T0074127

TELEHEALTH
SUCCESS

ADITI U. JOSHI, MD, MSC | BRANDON M. WELCH, MS, PHD

TELEHEALTH
SUCCESS

How to Thrive in the New Age of Remote Care

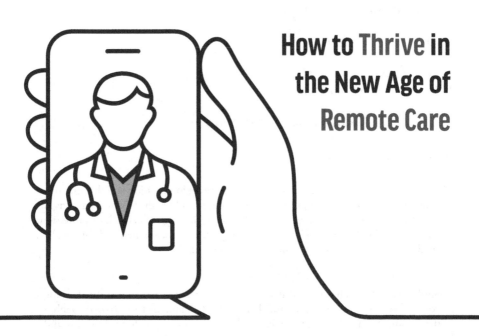

Forbes | Books

Published by Forbes Books, Charleston, South Carolina.

An imprint of Advantage Media Group.

Forbes Books is a registered trademark, and the Forbes Books colophon is a trademark of Forbes Media, LLC.

Printed in the United States of America.

10 9 8 7 6 5 4 3 2 1

ISBN: 979-8-88750-139-0 (Hardcover)
ISBN: 979-8-88750-140-6 (eBook)

Library of Congress Control Number: 2023910162

Book design by Analisa Smith.

This custom publication is intended to provide accurate information and the opinions of the author in regard to the subject matter covered. It is sold with the understanding that the publisher, Forbes Books, is not engaged in rendering legal, financial, or professional services of any kind. If legal advice or other expert assistance is required, the reader is advised to seek the services of a competent professional.

Since 1917, Forbes has remained steadfast in its mission to serve as the defining voice of entrepreneurial capitalism. Forbes Books, launched in 2016 through a partnership with Advantage Media, furthers that aim by helping business and thought leaders bring their stories, passion, and knowledge to the forefront in custom books. Opinions expressed by Forbes Books authors are their own. To be considered for publication, please visit books.Forbes.com.

Dedicated to the men and women who lost their lives caring for people with Covid.

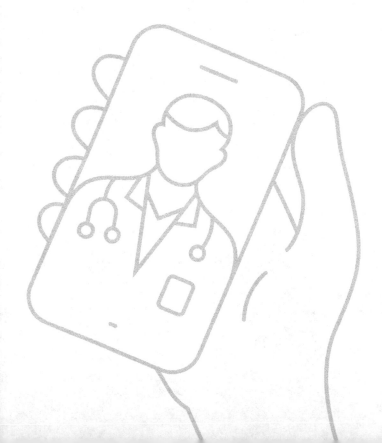

CONTENTS

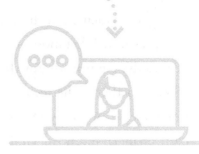

INTRODUCTION

Introducing Dr. Brandon M. Welch

I n late 2021, I ran into a physician colleague of mine. As we were catching up, the conversation naturally turned to his experience using telemedicine during the Covid-19 pandemic. (As the founder of Doxy.me, a telehealth technology company, I enjoy asking clinicians about their experience with telehealth.) My colleague had nothing but positive things to say about telemedicine. He talked about how much he and his patients enjoyed using it and how easy the software was to use. When I asked how much he'd been doing telemedicine since the pandemic, he said that once pandemic restrictions were lifted, administrators at his organization decided to go back to in-person care only. Given how pleased he and his patients had been during the pandemic, I was surprised by this decision.

I've been involved with telehealth for over a decade and have seen the value of it firsthand for its convenience, efficiency, and savings for patients and clinicians alike. Until this conversation, I had always assumed that most physicians shared my perspective, and that telehealth's continued growth was a matter of overcoming barriers. I believed that if the technology were easy to use, affordable, and unhampered by overly restrictive regulations, and if it came with a clear financial incentive, clinicians would use it.

Practically overnight, barriers telehealth had collectively struggled with for years disappeared, and Covid pushed the entire telemedicine field forward a decade. Thanks to emergency public health orders, the government was encouraging the use of telehealth, *and* providers were being reimbursed for it. Internet access was widely available, and telemedicine technology was, for the most part, affordable, widely accessible, and user friendly. During the pandemic, many clinicians and patients realized that telehealth isn't as challenging as they had once thought. As a result, telehealth utilization grew to *seventy-eight times* higher than before the pandemic.[1] As the CEO of Doxy.me, I personally witnessed telehealth sessions on the platform skyrocket from twelve thousand per day to nearly one million per day in under two months.

> **Covid pushed the entire telemedicine field forward a decade.**

However, I realized during my conversation with my colleague that all these advancements weren't enough to ensure telehealth's long-term adoption. He was far from alone; after the initial pandemic-era explosion in telehealth adoption, its utilization precipitously dropped before ultimately stabilizing at levels only *thirty-eight* times higher than before the pandemic.[1]

At the same time, I continued to hear clinicians and patients who were using telehealth successfully and wanted to use it more. As an associate professor at the Medical University of South Carolina, I found this dichotomy striking. What was the difference between those who no longer used telehealth and those who fully embraced it? I was particularly intrigued with adoption disparities among those coming from clinicians from the same specialty, background, and training. What could account for the difference? Why was one group able to recognize telehealth's value, overcome its inherent challenges, and ultimately find success, while the other merely tolerated it until they could go back to seeing patients in person? With my scientific curiosity piqued, it set me off in a new direction, and I dove into research.

My team and I reviewed thousands of research articles and publications on telehealth. We also conducted hundreds of hours of interviews with providers and administrators—both those who liked it and stuck with it, and those who had used and abandoned it. The explanation simply came down to one word: *success*. In essence, those who were *successful* using telemedicine continued to use it, and those who weren't abandoned it.

But what, exactly, does success mean in this context? Is it the same for everyone? After analyzing our results, we found that telehealth success can be grouped into five distinct domains:

1. *Patient success*: First and foremost, patients need to receive the quality of care they desire, in the way they prefer.

2. *Clinician success*: Clinicians and organizations need to provide quality care in a way that works best for them.

3. *Technology success*: Telehealth technology must work well and be easy to use.

4. *Financial success*: Clinicians, payers, and patients need to benefit financially from using telehealth.

5. *Compliance success*: Finally, clinicians need to not only stay out of legal trouble but also use healthcare laws and regulations to their advantage.

Importantly, we found that providers need to succeed *in all five* domains. There are many examples where clinicians were successful in some of the categories, but because they weren't successful in all of them, telehealth wasn't successful for them overall.

My team and I knew this information could help a lot of people and benefit the healthcare industry. Then came the hard part: summarizing and presenting the information so that others could benefit from it. We felt that a book would be the most effective way to deliver this information.

Though I have spent thousands of hours researching and developing telemedicine technology and have used it as a patient, I've never actually *provided* care by telemedicine. It would be disingenuous of me to tell clinicians how to successfully provide care by telehealth without actually having ever done it myself. With that in mind, I set out to find an experienced clinician who understood the ins and outs of caring for patients via telemedicine to help me write this book with an all-important clinical perspective.

Around this time, I met Aditi U. Joshi, MD, who was embarking on an independent telehealth consulting career. Aditi had already conducted thousands of virtual visits before the pandemic. And because of her extensive experiences with telehealth, she became a leader to her colleagues throughout the pandemic. She was clearly the perfect clinical partner to help write this book. Her experience, both as a clinician and health system administrator, is among the most extensive in the industry and has added immeasurable value and clinical experience to the topics we're here to present.

Introducing Dr. Aditi U. Joshi

By the time Covid hit, I had been working in telehealth for over seven years and had seen tens of thousands of virtual patients. I not only understood telehealth's potential, but as a former Assistant Medical Director of Doctors on Demand, I had heard every complaint and concern about it from health systems, patients, and other doctors. At the time, I was the Medical Director of Telehealth at Jefferson Health, a large academic center, running the direct-to-consumer (DTC) and tele-triage programs, staffed by me and a team of emergency medicine colleagues.

In early March of 2020, I was holed up in a hotel room attending a medical conference with a colleague, the assistant medical director of an ER, and our phones were ringing nonstop with requests for meetings, most of them regarding how to prepare for a full-scale pandemic. At a certain point we looked at one another, realized we were not going to make any of our conferences or meetings, jumped on a train, and headed back to Philadelphia. That was the beginning of the longest two weeks of my life.

As clinics, nonemergent procedures, and just about everything else ground to a halt, my telehealth team at Jefferson needed more than anything to rapidly scale our program to screen patients and order Covid tests for the tri-state area of Pennsylvania, New Jersey, and Delaware. Meanwhile, I watched the patient volume on our telehealth platform quickly increase to the point of overwhelm. At the time, I had only one other colleague on call. Until then, the clinic had never been so busy that one doctor was unable to handle the volume, but now it certainly was. I instantly knew that we wouldn't be able to handle this oncoming tidal wave on our own.

Like many other hospitals and clinics at the time, Jefferson turned to telehealth to screen and decrease Covid exposure. Fortunately, *unlike* most others at the time, we already had everything we needed: a tech platform, trained staff, an IT department on call, clinical pathways, telehealth training modules, and a quality assurance process. When I needed help with staffing, I could call on colleagues from other specialties to jump in and help, and because we used established telehealth training, processes, and protocols, the system worked efficiently.

Ten days after returning from the conference, I permitted myself a sigh of relief when I saw that our high patient volume was being handled by multiple doctors from multiple specialties, all of whom helped screen, coordinate testing, and care for patients. Ironically, despite running a virtual care program, I contracted Covid at the end of March and was subsequently bedridden for weeks.[2]

> **Years of preparing led to our success.**

With the benefit of hindsight, I can see that Jefferson's successful response to Covid began years before the pandemic hit. A concerted effort and a belief in telemedicine on the part of leadership and staff at Jefferson led to our ability to help thousands of people at a moment's notice. It took *years* of believing that there was an unexplored and untapped value in building virtual care, and that one day, there would be a time when it would be absolutely necessary. That day just came sooner, and in a more unexpected way, than any of us had initially anticipated. In the end, *being ready* led to our success.

Since 2020, we've seen telehealth's rapid expansion throughout the healthcare industry. Even though more patients and clinicians are doing telehealth than ever before, some myths, fears, and concerns stubbornly persist. Despite this expansion, I still hear some of the *same* fears today that I did a decade ago: that we cannot provide the same quality care virtually as in person, that patients don't necessarily want it, and that it will not be financially feasible.

I've been an emergency medicine doctor longer than I've been in telehealth, and much of my belief and commitment to telehealth technology stems from my experience working on the front lines. Writing this book brought back memories of working with fellow doctors; advocating and lobbying the government for policy changes; working with a small group of other telehealth believers on education, research, and telehealth expansion; dispelling myths in the media; and teaching my colleagues and students that technology was nothing to be afraid of.

Most vividly, I remembered my patients, both from the emergency department and those I saw via telehealth. Without them, I would never have learned what medicine today needs, what it can do, when it works best, or how awful it can be to struggle with access issues, how easy it is to go bankrupt without health insurance, and how desperately people want good healthcare for themselves and their families. I wanted to write this for them.

Today's healthcare system is facing serious challenges—the workforce is decreasing, costs are rising, and the American population is aging. Telehealth is a piece that can help with all of the above. When Brandon approached me to help write this book, it was a perfect opportunity to share why and how telehealth is and will continue to be crucial for patients, clinicians, and the broader healthcare system.

About This Book

We wrote this book to help healthcare stakeholders, clinicians, startups, and any organization working in healthcare to understand what it takes to be successful with telemedicine. The five success domains outlined in this book will give you a broad picture of where telehealth has been, where it still needs to go, and how you can make it work for you. Because the topics span broadly across healthcare, they will interest you whether you're a specialist at a large health system or a counselor running an independent practice.

The saying goes that "smart people learn from their mistakes, and wise people learn from others'." Following this principle, we'll make ample use of our personal experiences, those of others, and a veritable mountain of research and data. Again, our goal here is to help you be successful with telehealth, and with fewer missteps along the way.

Before we start in earnest, there are a few notes we want to convey up front. This book is not just about telehealth—it's about how to be *successful* with telehealth. As a result, we'll forgo some of the "What is telehealth?" kinds of topics you may find in other books in favor of focusing on the aspects of telehealth that directly influence success or failure. We assume you have a working knowledge of telehealth. Throughout the book, we'll use the words "telemedicine" and "tele-health" interchangeably to refer to the use of technology on the part of healthcare professionals who deliver care remotely.

Since telehealth is used by different types of healthcare professionals, doctors, nurses, specialists, and other providers, we don't want to inadvertently exclude anyone, so we are using the term "clinicians" to broadly represent any healthcare professional who provides care to patients, while occasionally specifying when required. While the content here is largely US-centric, most of the information we're here to share should be broadly applicable regardless of the country you call home. Finally, while Aditi is the principal narrator of the first two sections and half of the finance section, and Brandon will take the helm for majority of the rest, this book was a collaboration from start to finish, and we've both contributed significantly throughout.

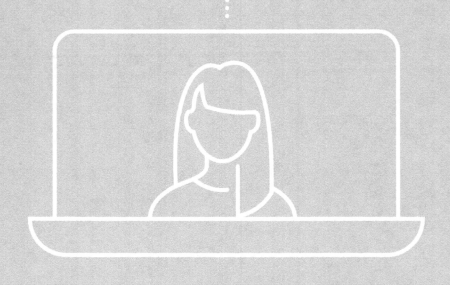

SECTION 1

Patient Success

Aditi U. Joshi

When medical students learn about the ideal physician, the first name to come up is often Dr. William Osler of Johns Hopkins, one of the founding fathers of modern medical education. One of his most important legacies is that of being a humanist; he taught his students that medicine is fundamentally the practice of dealing with and healing other humans. Despite Dr. Osler's then-revolutionarily humanistic approach, the institution of medicine has remained stubbornly paternalistic—one that *prescribes* treatment. Until quite recently, the patient hasn't had much of a voice. Though patients are the ultimate users of healthcare, their active involvement in the decision-making process has historically been relegated to the physician.

Until the midtwentieth century, when someone got sick, a family doctor would be summoned to the sick person's home, where he'd apply treatment, give his recommendations, collect his payment, and be on his way. Then, around the midtwentieth century, the pace of technological innovation within medicine accelerated rapidly. New devices allowed physicians to provide their patients with better care, but the complexity and cost of care made home visits impractical. Now, patients were increasingly traveling to hospitals and clinics within cities to receive care. This wasn't much of a problem for urban patients, but it made healthcare access more challenging for most everyone else.

Home visits were long thought to be a relic of the past until telehealth recently reintroduced them in a new, modern, twenty-first-century form. Today, telemedicine brings together the best of the past, present, and future by fostering a new, hybrid model of healthcare, one that combines the advanced technology within clinics and hospitals with more convenient, comfortable care at home. Telehealth increases not only access to healthcare but also its quality and efficiency. It turns out that involving patients in their care tends to improve clinician-patient relationships and their overall quality of care.

Ultimately, healthcare starts and ends with the patient, which is why we're starting this book in earnest with patients. To be successful with telehealth, *patients* must be successful, which requires that they're able to access care (chapter 1), receive quality care (chapter 2), and be satisfied with the care they receive (chapter 3).

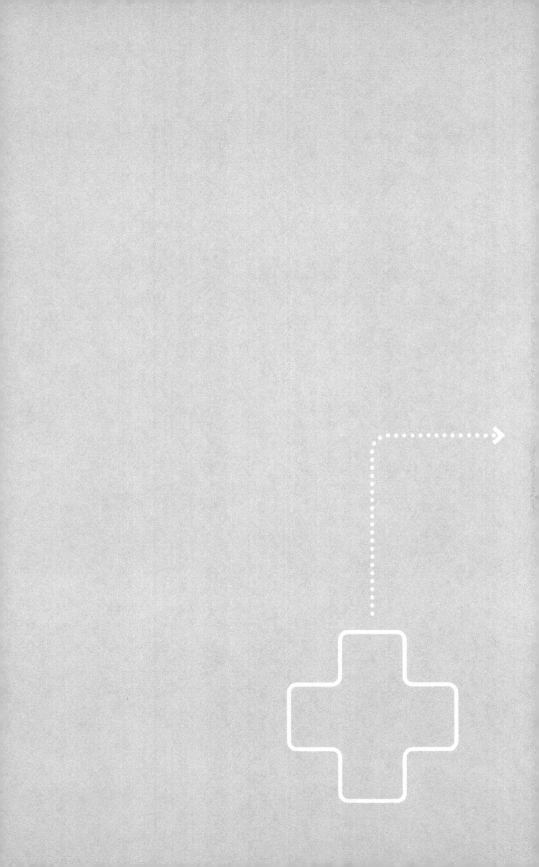

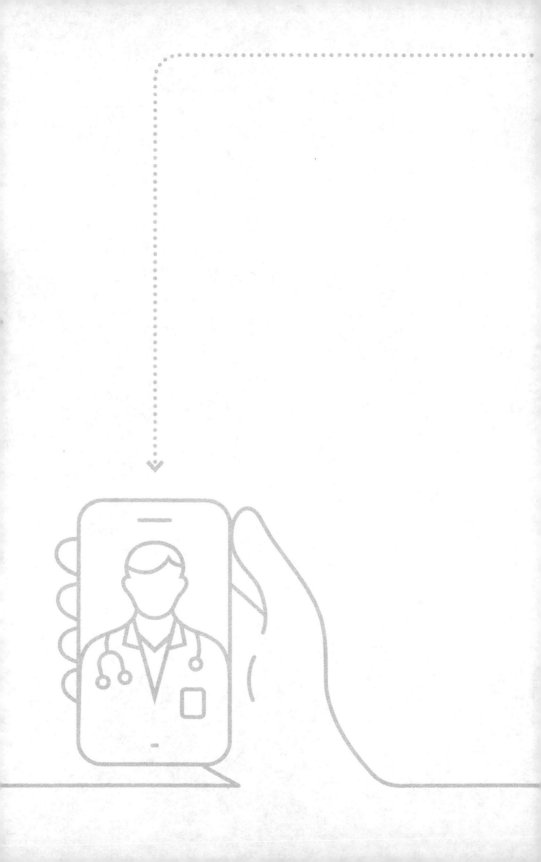

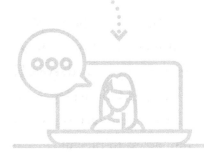

CHAPTER 1

Patient Access

While working at a rural clinic in the vast, dry, sparsely populated west coast of Australia, a forty-four-year-old nurse started having chest pain. He quickly recognized his symptoms as signs of an inferior STEMI, a blockage of the lower part of the heart, and one that accounts for 40 percent of all heart attacks.

Nearly a thousand miles from Perth, he knew he had no hope of getting to a catheterization lab within the recommended ninety minutes. He jumped on a video call with Emergency Telehealth Services (ETS), a telehealth program for rural care in Australia. With the help of their physicians and technicians, he placed his own IV, self-administered the first round of necessary medications, and began monitoring his vital signs. With ETS guidance, he placed his own defibrillator pads to give himself thrombolytics, which broke up the blood clots causing the heart attack. These actions collectively resolved his pain, stabilized his EKG changes, and bought him precious time.

Before long, he was picked up by the Royal Flying Doctor Service and transported by air to a cardiology unit in Perth. His coronary angiography showed severe blockage, so he was promptly treated with a stent, and ultimately lived to tell his tale. While his training gave him the necessary skills to administer self-care, telemedicine gave him access to the guidance of qualified professionals and ultimately extended his life.[3] Though not all examples of telehealth access are quite this dramatic, they're no less significant.

Healthcare access can be defined as the ability for patients to meet with a qualified health provider to obtain healthcare services—whether prevention, diagnosis, treatment, and/or management—within a reasonable period of time. After all, healthcare is only beneficial when it's accessible; the best, most efficient system in the world is worth little if no one can use it. There are many reasons patients are unable to access healthcare; they can be systemic, geographic, or social. Gender, income, sexuality, disability, race, age, and disease stigma all affect access to healthcare. Moreover, when these barriers overlap and an individual is part of more than one of these groups, it compounds and worsens the access issues.

Lack of access to healthcare is an enormous challenge for health systems worldwide, and a major contributor to poor health outcomes. Across the world, it is estimated that 5.7 million people in low- and middle-income countries die each year from poor-quality healthcare, and 2.9 million people die from being unable to access care.[4] From the start, telehealth has been touted as a solution to overcoming a variety of access barriers, and fortunately, telehealth has since shown that it *does* improve access to healthcare, principally by overcoming barriers that previously seemed formidable. Seventy-six percent of patients report that remote clinic visits made it possible for them to attend an appointment they would not otherwise have been able to.[5]

While telehealth hasn't completely removed every access barrier, it's done a tremendous amount of good in a short amount of time. In this chapter, we'll delve into common access barriers, and how telehealth can help overcome them.

Rural Care

The US is the fourth-largest country in the world by landmass, and 86 percent of it is considered rural. While roughly 20 percent of the US population lives in rural areas, only 10 percent of doctors do.[6] Given the scarcity of healthcare services in rural areas, rural patients have longer commute times, have fewer care options, don't visit doctors as regularly, receive less preventive care, and tend to present for care in the later stages of their diseases. As a result, rural patients experience worse health outcomes and higher death rates, higher rates of obesity, and higher rates of mental illness and addictive disorders.[7]

Furthermore, while urban tertiary care hospitals typically have in-house expertise for urgent care cases like stroke, heart attack, and trauma, most rural hospitals do not. As a result, clinicians at rural hospitals stabilize their patients before sending them on to a specialist at an urban center. As an attending physician at an urban tertiary care hospital, I've experienced this time and again. I'd typically have a brief phone call with a colleague at the rural hospital about the incoming patient and try to understand their workup and what specialty services they'd need—but I couldn't truly evaluate them until they arrived.

Sometimes I'd receive patients who had traveled two to four hours only to find that we could have cared for them remotely from their home hospital. I have seen numerous patients who didn't need our specialty services and have found myself repeatedly dismayed by the inefficiency and inconvenience. Telemedicine now allows us to evaluate rural patients and conduct a more thorough evaluation from a distance so we can better determine if they need to transfer, which has drastically improved the care and convenience for rural patients.

Telestroke is another urgent care use case making a positive impact on rural patients. Ten years ago, approximately 20 percent of American patients were not able to access timely stroke care. Today, with telestroke-capable emergency departments, a staggering 96 percent of people in South Carolina are now within one hour of life-saving stroke care.[8] Telestroke patients tend to be evaluated by stroke specialists and receive anticoagulants faster and require fewer time-consuming transfers, both of which lead to decreased mortality.[9]

> **With telehealth, distance is simply no longer the barrier it once was.**

Now, as just about anyone can access care that was previously available only in urban centers, rural patients are no longer required to travel long distances to receive care they need. Telehealth doesn't solely benefit rural patients seeking acute care; it's also used to increase access to care for rural patients from the convenience of home across many diseases, including mental health, orthopedics, HIV, and reproductive health.[10] With telehealth, distance is simply no longer the barrier it once was.

Specialist Access

Ironically, many modern access issues are in fact the consequence of *advances* in healthcare. Just a few generations ago, primary care doctors could address almost all of any given patient's needs. Back then, healthcare was simpler—a single doctor could do almost everything a patient could possibly need, from treating a cold to delivering a baby. In recent decades, with advancement in medical knowledge and technology, healthcare has become far more specialized. Today, there are nearly two hundred specialties and subspecialties to treat specific diseases. This isn't necessarily a bad thing; specialization has improved the quality of care for many diseases, and most patients are better as a result.

However, rampant specialization *has* made our interactions with the healthcare system more complicated. Most patients juggle multiple specialists and referrals, often leading to a breakdown in the continuum of care. Increasingly fragmented medical records can fail to provide a cohesive picture of a given patient's history. Most of the time, there isn't one single clinician taking ownership of a patient's care, which can lead to patients bouncing around between doctors, unnecessary extra visits, and repeat interventions. When multiple clinicians treat one patient without fully communicating, poor treatment quality, suboptimal outcomes, and higher costs often follow.

Telehealth can help solve the problems created by specialization and care fragmentation by improving communication and coordination between treating care providers. For example, a primary care physician and a specialist can collaborate over telehealth to develop a coordinated care plan for a patient, ensuring that all aspects of their care are integrated and consistent. This is particularly important for complex and critical cases involving multiple clinicians and care providers. Additionally, *provider-to-provider* telehealth, in which one doctor consults with a specialist physician about a patient over telehealth, is increasingly being used to overcome specialty access barriers. A number of telehealth companies, such as RubiconMD, provide primary physicians with on-demand remote access to specialists to provide expert guidance.

Another notable example of provider-to-provider telehealth is Project ECHO, which was launched in 2003 by liver disease specialist Sanjeev Arora, MD, who was frustrated that he could serve only a fraction of the hepatitis C patients in New Mexico. Because many patients with the disease were unable to travel long distances for specialty care at his clinic in Albuquerque, Dr. Arora created a free telehealth educational model to mentor community clinicians across the state on how to treat the disease. Project ECHO–trained community clinicians were ultimately found to be as good as the care provided by specialists, and the model has proven so successful that it's since been adopted across dozens of specialties in multiple countries.[11, 12]

Language and Communication

Not everyone speaks the same language; in fact, as many twenty-five million Americans have limited English proficiency, which leads to miscommunications between clinicians and patients.[13] Language barriers make it harder to access health services and to communicate with clinicians, which causes patients to avoid or delay care.[14, 15] Unsurprisingly, Americans with low English proficiency were found to experience high rates of medical errors and avoidable readmissions, as well as low rates of outpatient follow-up, use of preventive services, and medication adherence.[16]

Regardless, patients have a legal right to access healthcare services in their preferred language.[17] Informal translators, such as family members, often step in, but they're not ideal because important details can be left out or misunderstood, with potentially hazardous consequences. And while many interpreter services are available by telephone, the interpreter's ability to accurately read nonverbal cues is crucial to helping the patient and clinician fully understand one another. In-person, professionally trained, medicine-specialist interpreters are the best option available, but they come with higher costs, longer visits, and limited availability.[18]

Telehealth now allows clinicians to add an on-demand medically trained interpreter to video calls with their patients. Interpreter services like LanguageLine and Voyce integrate with telehealth apps to provide access to professional interpreters for hundreds of languages. In addition to being convenient and fast, video has the added benefit of allowing interpreters to observe nonverbal communication. Some clinicians are even starting to use telehealth interpreter services during in-person appointments due to their cost, efficiency, and availability. To be successful, telehealth software should also support multiple languages within its user interface, including text, buttons, and instructions; otherwise, they only perpetuate the language barriers that telemedicine can otherwise help to overcome.[19]

In addition to foreign languages, the deaf population is also an area of unique challenges and opportunities. Deaf Americans, for example, are less likely than the general population to effectively describe symptoms of strokes or heart attacks.[20] American Sign Language (ASL) interpreters help patients communicate their symptoms and ensure they understand what their clinician is telling them. While remote visits between clinicians, ASL interpreters, and deaf patients would not have been possible before telemedicine, 65 percent of deaf Americans still have communication challenges via telehealth despite the broad availability of interpreters.[20] In the meantime, real-time voice-to-text transcription, closed-captioning, and artificial intelligence that converts sign language to text will improve the remote care experiences of the deaf and hard of hearing.

Age

On a particularly busy telehealth shift during the pandemic, I had an eighty-five-year-old patient call in with their chief complaint listed as "Covid-19." This was before the national vaccine rollout, and the patient in question was in a high-risk age group, so I was fairly concerned. As our visit began, he cheerfully proceeded to tell me he had no symptoms or concerns; he simply wanted to set up a telehealth account, ensure he did everything correctly, and had the ability to connect to me in case he "needed me in the future." Aside from my relief that he was not presenting with Covid symptoms, I was charmed by his clear pride in figuring out the process for himself.

Because health concerns increase with age, the elderly are naturally higher consumers of healthcare than younger populations. Most face more formidable access barriers and struggle with additional issues: multiple chronic conditions, cognitive decline, mobility and transportation constraints, and the lack of social support and/or financial resources needed to receive quality care. Unsurprisingly, the elderly have the highest rates of morbidity and mortality. Moreover, as the number of older persons worldwide will double from 700 million in 2020 to 1.5 billion in 2050, these issues will continue to place a heavy burden on the healthcare system.[21]

> **One study found that telemedicine use actually increases with age.**

There are already many examples of telemedicine helping the elderly to age in place while continuing to receive the preventive, curative, and rehabilitative care they need across specialties.[22] Studies consistently find that telemedicine adoption is high and increasing among the elderly; [23] in fact, elderly patients are generally satisfied with telemedicine,[24] and one study found that telemedicine use actually *increases* with age.[25]

However, to ensure that telemedicine continues to benefit the elderly, it must be easy to use and accessible. Substantial barriers still exist; lack of equipment, limited technical literacy, and lack of assistance are most often cited as their chief barriers.[22] While the elderly do often have trouble with technology to the extent that they require assistance, it's not quite as bad as the pervasive stereotypes imply.[26] And in the end, some will always simply prefer to see their clinicians in person.[27]

It's not just the elderly patients to consider; each generation has its own healthcare preference peculiarities. Younger generations tend to seek digital options and preventive care, and they are least likely to have a primary care physician. Older populations value quality care and are the most likely to rely on their doctors' advice. Trust is important to them. Younger generations are a window of how healthcare is going to change and what telehealth will also need to provide. To be successful, telemedicine must be responsive to the preferences and needs of all ages, with an emphasis on convenience and usability.

Disability

Worldwide, approximately one billion people live with disabilities, which come in many forms: vision, movement, hearing, learning, communication, social, and mental. Disabilities can be due to a wide variety of physical and mental impairments—and generally limit one's ability to participate in normal activities. Those with disabilities are often the highest utilizers of healthcare, and their very disability can make it more challenging to access the care they need. Attending in-person medical visits is often a significant undertaking, particularly for patients with severe disabilities. While most healthcare facilities themselves are accessible, the added burden of traveling, coordinating, managing limited mobility, and ensuring safety make in-person care a challenge for disabled individuals and their caretakers.

Telemedicine can make it easier for those with disabilities to receive care. The first time I truly appreciated telehealth's benefits was by treating a young man who was paralyzed from the waist down, making it challenging for him to leave his house. He had a long history of bladder infections, which were so frequent that he readily recognized the symptoms. Ultimately, he was able to use telehealth in the middle of the night to get antibiotics for his infection without having to travel to his doctor's office.

Fortunately, remote patient monitoring and hospital-at-home programs are increasingly extending care to disabled patients' homes, and the ease of access helps homebound patients feel less isolated in seeking care. Features like live captioning, large text sizes, high-contrast displays, screen reader support, keyboard controls, remote control, group calling, and more all continue to help patients with disabilities. Going forward, it will be important to ensure that tele-health technology does not make it *harder* for disabled individuals to seek care. It's best to use telehealth technology that's easy to use and complies with the Americans with Disabilities Act.[28]

Racial and Ethnic Disparities

There can be no discussion of access in healthcare without talking about racial health disparities. Social stigma, lack of trust, cultural competence, prejudice, stereotyping, systemic racism, unconscious bias, and more all contribute to worse health outcomes for ethnic and racial minorities.[29] When compared to White counterparts, African

American, Hispanic and Native Americans experience higher rates of illness and death across a wide range of health conditions, whether diabetes, cancer, hypertension, obesity, asthma, or heart disease. They also have worse outcomes in terms of the care they receive and overall health expenditure. Racial disparities within healthcare are poor and have *worsened* in recent decades.[7]

Telehealth alone cannot solve this problem, but it's already making an impact. Telehealth reduced racial differences in appointment completion rates between White and Black patients.[30] Another study on musculoskeletal pain found that Black and Hispanic patients had greater improvements in clinical outcomes compared to White patients.[31]

Clinicians may not be familiar with a broad array of cultural beliefs, practices, or values, all of which can impact treatment plans and outcomes. Additionally, bias and discrimination in healthcare settings can lead to minority populations distrusting and being reluctant to use healthcare. Clinicians being culturally competent is imperative. One study demonstrated that having even one Black primary care physician in a county increased Black patients' life overall expectancy in that region.[32] There are already several telehealth services aimed at connecting patients with culturally similar physicians to reduce such racial and ethnic disparities. For example, Zocalo Health is working to improve virtual care to Latin populations, and MyBlackTelehealth facilitates appointments between African American patients and clinicians.

To be successful with telehealth, it's important to keep in mind how social determinants of health—including income, education, and insurance—affect minority patients and contribute to health disparities. Investigating why some of these disparities exist in the first place is the first step toward improving them.

Women's Health

Women have long suffered from a history of inequality that has always extended to healthcare. Around the world, many women and girls face significant barriers in terms of accessing healthcare: restrictions on mobility, lack of decision-making autonomy, restrictive laws, lower literacy rates, and domestic violence. Women are more likely than men to be uninsured and live in poverty. Gender bias causes clinicians to dismiss or downplay women's symptoms and concerns, resulting in delayed or incorrect diagnoses.[33] Historically, medical research has focused predominantly on men, resulting in a lack of understanding of how certain health conditions or treatments affect women. Finally, unpaid caregiving and childcare disproportionately fall on women, leading women to put the needs of family members above their own. All of these factors contribute to poorer health, chronic conditions, and compromised mental health.[33]

Again, telehealth alone cannot solve all of these problems, but it's already started to help. Women account for significantly more telehealth visits[34] and are more likely to choose telehealth than men.[35] Women accounted for 64 percent of general medical visits and sought out virtual behavioral healthcare at a higher rate. Women between the ages of 25 and 44 are also now the most frequent users of telehealth overall, while women between 45 and 64 are the most frequent users for chronic condition management. Women are also turning to telehealth for triage care for sick family members and their children to avoid trips to the doctor's office, and many report they would not have received care at all if telehealth services weren't available.[36]

Serving the needs of women is critical, and decreasing telehealth access would disproportionately impact women from accessing care overall. Already, a number of startups are offering telehealth services that cater to women. Maven, a virtual women's care company that offers a broad array of services, has already reached a $1 billion valuation. More niche companies like Carrot and Frame offer fertility services, Ruth Health offer postpregnancy recovery and lactation consulting, and others offer care for patients experiencing menopause.

Stigma and Disease

When doctors apply for a new medical license, depending on which state they are in, they may have to disclose whether they're currently being treated for mental health. For this reason, many are wary of getting mental health treatment. As a result, many prefer to pay for mental health services in cash without disclosing it. Sadly, stigma has contributed to the broader mental health crisis within the profession and has led to more physicians dying by suicide.[37]

Stigmatized patients in general are less likely to admit that they need help, seek healthcare services, and follow through with recommended treatments, all of which leads to delayed diagnosis and treatment. Some medical conditions are more stigmatized than others, including mental illness, substance abuse, sexually transmitted diseases, IBS, and visible skin conditions. Telehealth allows patients with stigmatized diseases to be treated more discreetly from a private location where exposure and embarrassment are avoided.

More than half of people with mental illness still don't receive treatment due to its stigma.[38] Telehealth reaches stigmatized patients who otherwise may not have sought treatment, such as mental health screening and prevention. In fact, mental health is now one of the most popular uses of telehealth; 36 percent of patients with mental health or addiction disorders use telehealth services.[39]

Many patients are simply more comfortable discussing sensitive issues through a telehealth platform than in a face-to-face setting. I've seen plenty of these cases myself, whether it's teens asking about sexual health, patients concerned about their alcohol intake, or those who are curious as to what constitutes a medical diagnosis of depression. All were able to confidently ask me questions over video, where in the past they may have resorted to asking friends or Google.

Telehealth also makes it easier for stigmatized patients to connect with others in online support groups that bring together people with shared diseases for mutual support, whether by sharing their experiences of depression or taking a particular medication for HIV. In general, telehealth helps patients feel more connected, less alone, and able to share and receive the information they need.

> **In general, telehealth helps patients feel more connected, less alone, and able to share and receive the information they need.**

Access to healthcare is a challenge for many and comes in different forms, none of which exists in a vacuum. While telemedicine has helped overcome some access issues, patient access remains a huge cause of disparity in global healthcare. We could devote entire additional chapters to other access issues, including those experiencing homelessness or barriers imposed by religion, culture, sexuality, economics, immigration status, and beyond. To be successful with telemedicine, clinicians must recognize the systemic and social barriers their patients face and then tailor their telemedicine program accordingly to overcome them. All can, and should, benefit from telehealth.

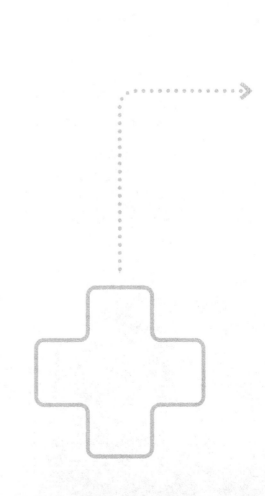

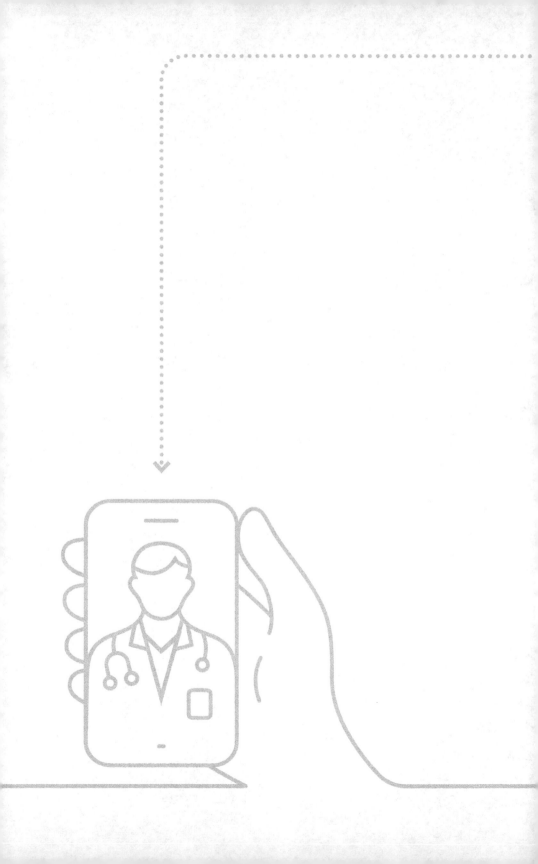

CHAPTER 2

Quality of Care

A forty-two-year-old woman experiencing homelessness with a history of uncontrolled diabetes and substance use was in the ER one summer day. Up until that point, the ER had been the patient's only source of healthcare, not allowing her chronic conditions to be adequately cared for, nor adequately addressing her social needs. Upon her discharge, a community health worker from Pair Team, a telehealth company helping to improve care to Medicaid-applicable patients, noted that she would benefit from their support, which they call Whole Person Care.

After providing her with a baseline assessment and support with food and housing, Pair Team also connected her to a nurse practitioner by video for help with her diabetes. Telehealth was used throughout her program for check-ins and acute care. When she was unsure whether she needed to visit the ER, she conferred with her nurse practitioner by video, who was often able to manage her case remotely. Despite a number of harrowing subsequent events, including her tent being removed by the city, an unanticipated ER visit, and almost falling out of the Pair Team program, she was ultimately able to improve her health. In fact, within six months, she quit smoking, lost weight, improved her blood sugar levels, and rebuilt family relationships. This is an inspiring example of using telehealth to provide quality, patient-centered care.

> **For telehealth to be successful, the quality of care delivered has to be as good or better than in-person care.**

Quality care is defined by the World Health Organization (WHO) as care that is safe, effective, and people-centered, delivered in a timely, equitable, and efficient way.[40] High-quality care is the primary objective of any good healthcare system. Poor-quality care not only affects individuals, but also families, communities, and the population as a whole. For instance, relatively straightforward improvements to the quality of care could reduce maternal and neonatal deaths by 28 percent and decrease stillborns by 22 percent in many countries around the world.[41]

Various government agencies and accreditation organizations such as the Agency for Healthcare Research & Quality and The Joint Commission establish guidelines and support initiatives to help clinicians establish and maintain quality care. The ultimate objective is to close the gap between what's considered the standard for good healthcare and the healthcare that people actually receive.

For telehealth to be successful, the quality of care delivered via telehealth has to be as good or better than in-person care. With that in mind, this chapter will explore patient safety, effectiveness, and people-centered care in the context of telehealth.

Patient Safety

In 1999, when the Institute of Medicine (IoM) released a report about patient safety called *To Err Is Human*, it sent shock waves through the medical industry. The report estimated that as many as ninety-eight thousand people die in any given year from medical errors including treatment, surgical, diagnostic, and medication errors, as well as hospital-acquired infections.[42] Fortunately, the report was a catalyst for change. Two years later, the IoM published *Crossing the Quality Chasm,* which highlighted activities that have since significantly improved patient safety: an increased emphasis on implemented protocols and checklists, improved training for staff on how to identify and reduce risks and hazards, the establishment of adherence to standard operating procedures and precautions, the use of computer-guided clinical decision support, and greater patient education and monitoring.[43] Twenty-six Patient Safety Indicators (PSI) have since become a standard way of measuring rates in which an adverse event occurs per thousand patients, and in turn, patient safety has increased overall. For example, blood-borne infections decreased by 43 percent and Methicillin-resistant Staphylococcus aureus (MRSA) by 22 percent.[44]

Given the importance of patient safety, it's not surprising that clinicians and administrators have always been concerned about the safety of telehealth in particular. (My physician colleagues were particularly concerned about performing full physical exams remotely.[a]) Again, for telehealth to be successful, it has to be as safe or safer than in-person care. Fortunately, several studies have demonstrated that telehealth *is* as safe as in-person care. In a cohort study of over one million primary care patients, those who had telehealth visits had significantly lower medication prescriptions and orders and no differ-

---

a   We discuss this issue more in the clinician section.

ence in adverse health events, including emergency department visits or hospitalizations.[45]

At the beginning of Covid, ophthalmologists wanted to determine whether it was safe to triage their emergency patients via telehealth. They compared two groups, each with over four hundred patients, the first in person, and the second via telehealth. Despite *twice* as many patients returning to use tele-triage compared to in-person triage—possibly due to convenience—the tele-triage group required fewer specialist reviews, and the rate of harm was 0 percent.[46]

In a recent randomized clinical trial of patients receiving hospital-level acute care at home, daily in-home physician visits were compared to daily remote telemedicine visits. In testing for infection, heart failure, chronic obstructive pulmonary disease, and asthma, researchers found that remote care had a rate of 6.9 of 100 adverse events[b] compared to 3.8 for in-person care. Though telehealth had a higher rate of adverse events, the number was not outside the normal range, and the authors of the study concluded that remote care was noninferior in terms of safety to in-person care.[47]

In certain circumstances, telehealth can also be potentially *safer* than in-person care. Paradoxically, the hospital is simultaneously the most and least safe place to be while sick. The pandemic made this clear to all, as it was far safer to get care at home rather than be potentially exposed to Covid in public. Even outside of global pandemics, hospital-acquired infections (HCAIs) are a major concern for admitted patients. For those with compromised immune systems, telehealth can significantly decrease the risk of hospital- or clinic-acquired infections. Nearly 1.7 million hospitalized patients annually acquire HCAIs while being treated for other health issues, and an astonishing one in seventeen die as a result.[48]

---

b   Defined here as pressure injury, delirium, and falls.

In my experience, providing in-person care can be more distracting than telehealth. When I first began doing telehealth consults in 2013, the extent to which it spared me from constant interruptions, calls, and distractions typical of any emergency department came as a surprise. My telehealth encounters were truly one-on-one. Because patients had my undivided attention, I could make sure they understood their treatment plan and disease progression and had time to comprehensively answer all of their questions.

Granted, there are situations where telehealth can be less safe than in-person care. A key study among patients and providers identified several situations where telemedicine was felt to be inappropriate, including patients with severe conditions, situations where a physical examination is necessary for a diagnosis, and visits for procedures that can only be done in person such as vaccinations.[49] A review of tele-mental health sources identified suicidality, domestic abuse, and eating disorders as the three main areas where telehealth should be provided with extreme caution. With suicidality and domestic abuse, the risk of harm can be imminent and difficult to assess remotely, and for eating disorders, it's easier for clients to hide certain behaviors remotely.[50] If you encounter these situations as a provider during a telehealth visit, refer the patient in question for in-person care, and when these situations are unavoidable, have an emergency plan in place.

Effective Healthcare

On December 14, 1799, George Washington began to experience chest congestion and a sore throat after being exposed to cold, wet conditions. His personal physician of forty years, Dr. James Craik, responded with a battery of then-common treatments: bloodletting;

an enema; a concoction of molasses, butter, and vinegar; and a toxic tonic that caused his throat to blister. Doctors at the time generally believed these remedies would draw the "bad humours" out of his blood. They failed to work, and the nation's first president died that evening.

There's no benefit to receiving healthcare if it doesn't work; at best, it's a waste, and at worst, it's dangerous. Healthcare has come a long way since eighteenth-century medicine, but ineffective healthcare persists today. For this reason, effectiveness—the ability of an intervention to have a meaningful effect on patients—is one of the main tenets of care quality. Effectiveness also refers to doing the right things to achieve a desired outcome. Today, the "right thing" principally refers to making healthcare decisions based upon the best available evidence and clinical expertise—what is referred to as "evidence-based care."

Clinical researchers generate the evidence, often through clinical trials, as to whether a certain treatment is as or more effective than another. Professional organizations and governments then create protocols and guidelines to help clinicians make correct, evidence-based decisions. In the end, it's largely up to the clinician to provide effective, evidence-based care to their patients. As such, it is natural for clinicians to wonder whether the care provided over telehealth is effective. Or to put it another way: can clinicians provide evidence-based care over telehealth? The answer ultimately comes down to outcomes. Do patients get better, stay the same, or get much worse?

Fortunately, there have already been a number of illuminating studies on this subject. One systematic review of neurosurgery patient management found telemedicine to be successful in 99.6 percent of cases. Four out of five telemedicine failures were due to technology failure; the remaining were due to patients requiring further face-to-face evaluation or treatment.[51] Another large-cohort study involving half a million test subjects compared quality performance measures for primary care patients exposed to telemedicine versus in person using the Healthcare Effectiveness Data and Information Set (HEDIS); it found that telemedicine had significantly *better* performance scores in eleven of sixteen quality measures, no statistical difference on three, and was worse on two.[52]

In particular, the telemedicine group was unanimously better than in-person care at testing-based (e.g., a cardiovascular (CVD) panel and diabetes testing) and counseling-based measures (e.g., cancer screening, mental health screening, tobacco intervention). In turn, the medication-based quality measures (e.g., antiplatelet medicine and antibiotic stewardship) were modestly better for in-person care. As this study shows, quality of care over telehealth is not only as good, but often *better* than in-person care.

There are a variety of other useful clinical measures that can be used to evaluate effectiveness. For instance, a 2019 meta-analysis of randomized clinical trials between in person and telemedicine diabetes care found greater reduction in HgBA1C, the measure of blood sugar levels in diabetics, in the telemedicine groups. Interestingly, older patients, as well as treatments lasting longer than six months, performed significantly better with telemedicine,[53] and other diabetes research has further shown improved adherence and lower A1C using telehealth.[54]

Effectiveness can also be measured by comparing diagnostic accuracy between telehealth and in-person care. The Mayo Clinic studied new patients without previous histories who were seen on telehealth for new complaints and then followed up with them in person. In the end, researchers found that the clinicians got the right diagnosis correct over telehealth 87 percent of the time—impressive, especially given that all the patients in the study hadn't previously been seen by the attending clinician.[55]

Patient adherence to prescribed treatment is also an important component of effectiveness. Here, the results have been encouraging as well. A pilot study on using telehealth to provide cognitive behavioral therapy to treat African American women with HIV was as effective as in-person care at improving antiretroviral therapy adherence and depression symptoms.[56] Similarly, several diabetes studies show that telemedicine had a positive impact on adherence to blood glucose monitoring, day-to-day self-care decision-making, and adherence to medications.[53]

Healing is another critical component of effective outcomes. Recovering at home consistently leads to better recovery times than at hospitals, perhaps because there is less exposure to infections, lower stress levels, family support, and the opportunity to simply get better sleep.[57] Telehealth shows enormous promise because it allows patients to remain at home while they recover. A 2020 analysis found telemedicine to have no significant differences in wound healing compared to standard treatment for wound care and earlier interventions.[58]

Readmissions, when a patient gets worse and has to go *back* to their hospital, are a standard quality benchmark of the quality of care and are a factor in reimbursement. While some readmissions are a result of unavoidable health complications, others are avoidable. Telehealth has shown either no difference or has significantly reduced readmission for heart failure, postoperative care, and other chronic heart diseases. A study on cancer-related surgeries found no difference in ninety-day readmission rates between telemedicine and in-person postoperative visits.[59] In another study of discharged heart failure patients, those who received telemedicine visits were less likely to be readmitted to the hospital within thirty days compared to patients who received no follow-up care.[60] When telehealth is used as part of a plan that includes check-ins, remote monitoring, education, and interventions, the results are more dramatic; several studies among discharged heart failure patients consistently saw decreases in thirty-day readmissions rates, from about 20 percent to under 6 percent.[61, 62]

In emergency care, the results are less promising. A recent study on emergency department patients showed patients who had telehealth follow-up had *more* returns to the hospital than those who followed-up in person.[63] The study's authors noted many possible reasons for this, including the inherent limitations of clinicians to physically examine patients, as well as the rural location of patients in the telemedicine group seeking care. Some of those reasons were not about acute care, reinforcing that standardizing telehealth guidelines may improve its effectiveness. The bottom line is that while telemedicine has been shown to be as effective or more effective than in-person care, it isn't always. Where it isn't, clinicians should stick with in-person care and keep in mind that telehealth is an invaluable *supplement* to in-person care.

> **Telemedicine allows patients to meet with clinicians sooner.**

Timeliness is important to achieving effective healthcare. Geriatric patients have higher mortality depending on the timeliness of consultation.[64] In an analysis of cancer patients, even a week-long delay tripled the odds of patients dying.[65] Telemedicine generally allows patients to meet with clinicians sooner. One study found that telehealth reduced the time to seeing an emergency physician by six minutes, and at a time when every second counts.[66] Another 2021 systematic review on pediatric telemedicine found that patients were both seen and that their life-saving procedures commenced sooner.[67] DTC telehealth also generally leads to patients being seen faster, both for treatment and obtaining necessary information.[68]

Patient-Centered Care

Patient-centered care is about being responsive to the individual patient and their health goals, values, and preferences in a way that empowers patients and providers to make decisions *together*. Over the last few years, there has been increased recognition of including patients' wants, needs, and goals regarding care delivery. After all, not all patients may have the same goals. A chronic obstructive pulmonary disease (COPD) patient may have the goal of going for a short walk, while another patient may be training for a marathon. Encouragingly, research increasingly shows that taking into account patient values, preferences, wants, and needs results in improved satisfaction, better resource allocation, decreased costs, and also better clinician productivity.

Telehealth is a great venue for having these conversations because it offers convenience and timeliness and increases the ease of care coordination. Providing care often involves the input of one or more family members, and conducting group telehealth calls to discuss a care plan with everyone involved makes the process more inclusive and patient centered. Most patient-centered care models include shared decision-making, understanding patient/family preferences and values, and sharing information to foster making informed decisions, all of which make patients and their families part of the care team. Patient-centered care for telehealth patients has also shown success in increasing patients' feelings of satisfaction.[69] In heart failure patients, having control and information led to feelings of safety and generally feeling closer to their care team.[70]

Care navigators—who help patients find the services they need, explain things in ways they understand, and provide the support people need to get better—play a crucial role here. They're increasingly turning to telehealth to help them do their jobs better. In a diabetic monitoring program, for example, nurse interventionists monitored patients, which led to improved blood glucose control, high rates of adherence, and high patient satisfaction.[71]

Sometimes patient-centered care goes beyond what a professional can provide, and many patients are compelled to turn to other patients or support groups for answers. Through video conferencing, patients with certain diseases can attend group counseling or connect with other patients with the same diagnosis to provide emotional and social support, often reducing feelings of anxiety, isolation, and loneliness.[72]

Being responsive to patient needs and desires requires clinicians to understand how their care affects patients from their patients' perspectives. In turn, an increasing number of clinical research studies are using patient-reported outcome measures (PROMs) to measure how telemedicine affects health-related quality of life, adherence, and emotional functioning.[73] PROMs are also used to assess patient perspective during treatment. One study among cancer patients using telehealth had higher rates of PROM survey completion rates compared to in-person care.[74]

Quality of care relates to more than just clinical outcomes—it must also consider quality of life. Quality-adjusted life-year (QALY) can help determine whether care improves or worsens someone's daily life in terms of their ability to carry out the activities of daily life; this measure includes freedom from pain and mental disturbance. QALYs are calculated by estimating the years of life remaining after a particular intervention and then weighting each year with a quality-of-life score on a 0–1 scale. For telephone-based ulcer treatment in India and Bangladesh,[75] retinopathy treatment in Singapore and New York City,[76] and for rheumatoid arthritis in Europe,[77] telemedicine contributed to 13.1, 14.66, and 0.7 quality adjusted life years respectively, demonstrating utility around the world.

Patients are entitled to receive safe, effective, patient-centered healthcare. Telehealth has demonstrated that quality of care is possible in a number of scenarios; in most use cases, it either improves or shows no inferiority to in-person care. While there are some gaps, when used properly, telehealth can deliver care as good as or better than in-person care. To be successful with telemedicine, ensure you're able to safely provide care to patients remotely, and strive to make your care more effective and to be responsive to your patients' health goals.

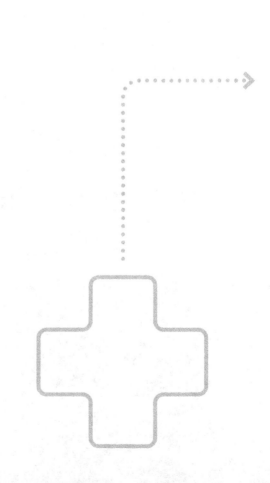

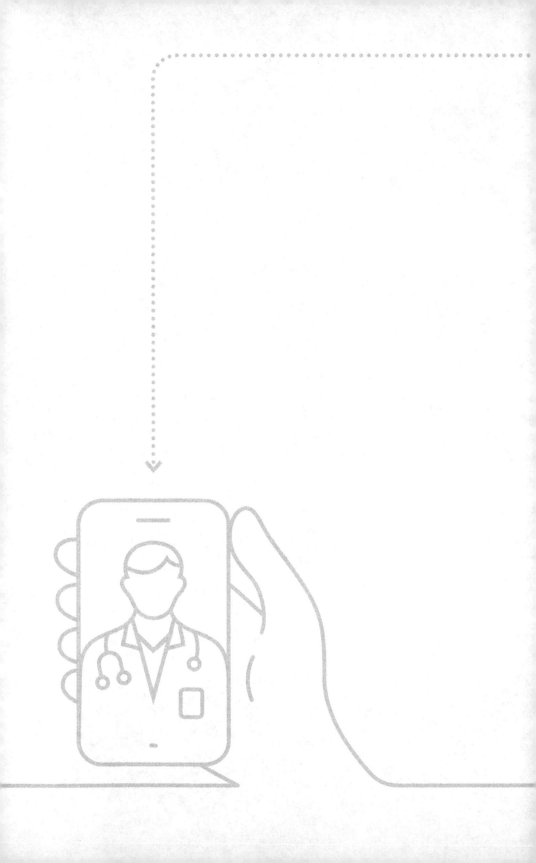

Patient Experience

I 've seen about twenty-five thousand telemedicine patients in my career. Early on, few wanted to use telemedicine, though more often than not, they simply didn't know what it was. When I did put the practice in place, many of my first-time telemedicine patients came away from the interaction grateful for the information and care they received *and* surprised by the ease of the process. A mom at the beach was able to stay outdoors rather than having to take her kid into their doctor's office. A woman who was traveling and ran out of her meds was happy to get a refill from afar. My favorite response of all was from a patient who, after calling in on the recommendation of a family member, concluded our interaction by saying, "I can't believe you're a real doctor. I thought this was some sort of scam."

Early on, telehealth engagement was largely a chicken and egg problem. Clinicians didn't use it and assumed patients didn't want it, so they didn't offer it. Meanwhile, patients didn't know it was possible or think it was safe, so they didn't ask for it. That made clinicians continue to avoid using it, and from there, round and round it went. Many early direct-to-consumer telehealth companies invested considerable time and resources to demonstrate that telehealth visits were convenient and trustworthy. At Doctor on Demand, we tried a number of initiatives to educate people and allowed them to try it for free. We made TV appearances and spoke to famous parenting blog hosts to drum up interest. Our efforts worked to an extent, but nothing got patients to use telehealth more than Covid.

Again, telehealth success begins and ends with the patient experience. The more your patients experience the benefits and conveniences of telehealth, the more they'll grow to love it and prefer to use it. Conversely, the more patients have poor experiences, the more they'll avoid it. There are several factors that contribute to patient satisfaction and preference for telemedicine. In this chapter we'll examine the features patients like and dislike in telemedicine, and how their responses influence their desire to use it—or not.

Patient Satisfaction

The terms "patient experience "and "patient satisfaction" are often used interchangeably, but they're not the same. By evaluating both patient satisfaction and patient experience, clinicians can gain a more complete understanding of the quality of care they're providing.

In essence, patient *experience* is a comprehensive measure of a patient's healthcare experience and includes several aspects of healthcare delivery that patients value highly: timely appointments, convenience, ease of access, and quality interactions. Patient experience is typically assessed through surveying and interviewing patients. For example, Centers for Medicare & Medicaid Services (CMS) uses the Hospital Consumer Assessment of Healthcare Providers and Systems (HCAHPS) to understand patient experience by asking recently hospitalized patients about their stays. In 2022, one of their surveys noted that patients found telehealth visits more positive than in-person care and that patients found doctor communication to be better on video.[78] Similar results subsequently presented across a variety of specialties.[79]

Patient *satisfaction* is concerned with how patients evaluate the *quality* of their healthcare experience. It is increasingly being assessed in surveys as a marker of quality of care, and relates to access, relevance to need, effectiveness, and efficiency. To assess patient experience, one must find out from patients themselves whether something that should've happened in a healthcare setting actually happened—and how often. *Satisfaction* relates to whether the patient's *expectations* were met. This can mean many things and can uncover previously obscured flaws in the system.

A considerable number of peer-reviewed studies con-

> **A considerable number of peer-reviewed studies consistently show that patients are satisfied with telemedicine.**

sistently show that patients are satisfied with telemedicine; in fact, the vast majority are seeing satisfaction rates of 80 percent or greater.[80, 81] Patient satisfaction with telehealth even remained high throughout the years before Covid, across multiple specialties and countries.[82] It remained high during the pandemic—sometimes higher than in-person care.[83]

There are a number of reasons for this. First, going to see a provider in person can be an inconvenient, time-consuming endeavor; it tends to require busy patients taking time off from work or school, traveling to the doctor's office, and sitting in a waiting area for an often unspecified amount of time. Chris and Alicia LaBonne discovered this when their seven-year-old daughter was diagnosed with a Wilms' tumor.[84] Instead of having to drive over two hours to the nearest specialty center in Nashville every two weeks, they were able to see their pediatric oncologist online. Chris was spared having to take an entire day of work to travel while continuing specialty care, and thankfully, their daughter fully recovered. Many other families similarly continue to benefit from remote cancer care; one study estimates that telehealth saves cancer patients between $147 and $186 per visit in travel savings and reductions in lost productivity.[85]

Unsurprisingly, long wait times in particular are negatively associated with patient satisfaction, and convenience was one of the biggest advantages of telemedicine promoted by early advocates. A colleague once told me his patients loved telemedicine because they didn't have to fight for parking or navigate the complicated design of his hospital and could go about their work or household chores as they waited for their calls to start. My colleague's patients aren't alone. One study demonstrated a 95–100 percent patient satisfaction rate with telemedicine and found the main reasons to be convenience, decreased travel time, and cost.[86] Another systematic review found that travel savings represented the most important advantage of having a virtual consultation, followed by time savings, cost savings, and reduced family interruption.[83]

Telemedicine is also associated with shorter waiting times in general. An analysis of over eight hundred postop virtual visits showed wait times of 3.8 minutes, whereas the national average in-person wait time was 18.5 minutes.[87] Another meta-analysis of telehealth trials for outpatient cancer care found telehealth wait time was twenty-nine minutes shorter compared to in-person care.[88]

Today, patients generally expect telehealth to be more convenient to use rather than less—nine out of ten find telehealth to be more convenient than in-person visits.[89] As a result, I've sometimes found that patients get frustrated upon learning that they'll need to schedule an in-person visit when their initial expectation was to *only* use telehealth. This is understandable to an extent; going to the doctor can be an uncomfortable experience for patients for a variety of reasons. Some feel anxious, fearful, or stressed because of negative past experiences. Others have a general fear of medical procedures, and the rest may feel embarrassed or stigmatized about seeking medical attention for their conditions.

Receiving care in a comfortable environment tends to make people feel safer and more open to asking questions, and home is often a more comfortable place for patients than a clinic. Correspondingly, 88 percent of patients rated their comfort level seeing a doctor via telemedicine as a ten out of ten.[90] Telehealth also makes it easier to bring in family members, interpreters, and other care advocates, all of whom tend to increase patient comfort levels.

There are, however, some cases where patients feel *less* comfortable using telehealth—lack of experience with technology and a general distrust of the security and privacy of digital systems tend to be the biggest culprits.[91] Fortunately, practice helps; several months of using telehealth has been found to have a significant correlation with increased comfort in using it.[92]

It's important to note that *whom* the patient sees via telemedicine dramatically impacts patient comfort. A study led by Brandon in 2016, when only 3.5 percent of surveyed patients had used telemedicine, more than half were nevertheless willing and comfortable with seeing their established primary care provider virtually.[93] When the same survey was repeated in 2022, even higher feelings of willingness, comfort, and satisfaction were revealed compared to the 2016 study.

CLINICIAN-PATIENT RELATIONSHIP

One of the biggest factors of patient satisfaction is the quality of the clinician-patient relationship. Its importance simply cannot be overstated. Patients who feel heard, respected, and cared for by their providers are more comfortable discussing their health concerns, as well as more likely to follow the advice of clinicians they trust. Traditionally, the clinician-patient relationship is established in person, face to face, while sharing the same physical space. Without these time-honored elements at their disposal remotely, most clinicians wonder how telehealth will impact the clinician-patient relationship and whether it can be established and maintained as effectively as in person.

Fortunately, most relationship building doesn't require physical presence, but it *does* require active listening, empathy, respect, trust, education, and follow-up—all of which can occur by telemedicine. In fact, a survey of social workers found they were surprised at how strong a connection they could foster remotely, and during the pandemic, they also noted that it was safer, because they could see patient's facial expressions without a mask being required.[94] Of the many studies that look at the impact of telemedicine on the clinician-patient relationship, most suggest that success is founded upon trust and communication, all of which patients still manage to receive via telehealth.

The doctor-patient relationship starts with a foundation of trust; studies have shown that higher physician trust is associated with higher patient satisfaction with telemedicine.[95] Convenience, time spent, and cost all additionally had a significant impact on trust,[95] though some studies also show that patients find that comfort and trust vary depending on context.[96] For instance, patients remain less willing and comfortable having a telemedicine call with a clinician they do not know,[93] and they would rather wait to see their own tele-health doctor than a new one. [97] Surgery patients in particular found more comfort and trust via in-person consultations.[98]

Effective communication is essential to the provider-patient relationship. On top of contributing to trust and comfort, it also ensures that patients understand their clinician clearly, which helps them make informed decisions about their care. Crucially, one pandemic-era study found that 86 percent of patients and 95 percent of clinicians felt they were able to communicate what they needed over telehealth,[99] and in another, 93 percent of telemedicine users rate their doctors ten out of ten in terms of explaining their condition in an easily understood manner.[90]

Telemedicine enables effective communication in a large part simply by making it easier and more convenient for both clinicians and patients to meet and talk. Again, I was surprised by the lack of distraction on telehealth calls versus seeing patients in person within a busy emergency department. For patients, meeting from home can be more distracting or less, depending on the environment.[100] Time spent is an all-important attribute of communication, and because telehealth allows comparably distractionless visits, the visits are often shorter than they would have been in person, while accomplishing the same things.[101]

The ability for patients to talk to an attentive provider about their concerns is often relief enough. I once met a patient over tele-health who had just had abdominal surgery and developed severe shoulder pain. After some questions, I realized that she'd had laparo-scopic surgery, and one of the common but nonobvious aftereffects is shoulder pain from diaphragmatic irritation. While her pain persisted, her relief at finding an explanation for her pain from a trusted source was obvious. Telehealth made finding that answer easy and saved her an unnecessary trip to urgent care.

Bad news is often the toughest communication for clinicians to deliver—and for patients to receive. There has been a good deal of discussion about the extent to which clinicians can and should deliver bad news over telehealth; during the pandemic doctors had little choice.[102] Oncologists receive particularly extensive training in delivering bad news and had to adapt to doing so via telemedicine throughout the pandemic like everyone else. Much of what they did revolved around connecting with patients without the ability to touch, as well as in managing interruptions.[103]

Patients are generally divided on this issue. At a hospital in Scotland, about half of cancer patients did not want to hear bad news over telemedicine,[104] and if they did, they wanted a specialist nurse present.[105] Yet in a different study within palliative medicine, 64 percent *preferred* to hear bad news over video, or had no preference at all.[106] In the end, patients who like telemedicine in general may simply be more willing to hear bad news virtually, as a study of neuromuscular patients found.[92]

If done improperly, telehealth can have a negative impact on the clinician-patient relationship, but technical issues tend to be the biggest deterrent to satisfaction,[107] a topic we will later devote a section to. Overall, given the quality of the patient-doctor connection and the ease of use, patients generally have a very high level of satisfaction with telemedicine.[96]

Preference

While a patient may have had a positive, satisfactory experience with telemedicine, it doesn't mean they'll always choose it. Healthcare in the US remains a free market with many options, so patients can find another provider if and when they're not satisfied. As a result, clinicians need to be responsive to their patients. With that said, a positive experience and high satisfaction increase the likelihood that a patient will return. Several studies show that a strong majority of patients came away from telehealth encounters

> **A positive experience and high satisfaction increase the likelihood that a patient will return.**

satisfied and would use it again in the future,[95, 108, 109] and one found that 85.8 percent would "strongly recommend" telemedicine to others.[110] Patients also reported that they would be "very likely" to use telehealth services to refill medications, prepare for upcoming visits, review test results, and receive education. Unsurprisingly, prior experience with telemedicine increases the likelihood of preferring to use it in the future.[111]

Cost, of course, strongly influences patient preference, and will forever be a huge determinant. Patients like telehealth even more when they find out that it's generally cheaper,[110] and if in-person care costs more, telemedicine preference increases compared to when cost was not a factor.[112] The "who factor" again plays a role here: patients who saw their own doctor via telehealth were more likely to feel like their telehealth visit was comparable to an in-person visit, would use telehealth again, and would be willing to pay the same for telehealth as an in-person visit.[113]

While several studies have found that patients are ready and willing to use telemedicine, some generally prefer in-person care overall, particularly when the process of obtaining it is complicated.[112] Others refer to the difficulty of fostering a personal connection remotely.[81]

More specifically, patients generally view physical examinations and diagnostic tests as most precise, accurate, and thorough when done in person.[114] Patients also prefer to be in person when receiving a new diagnosis or when a physical evaluation is necessary.[92] As a result of these preferences, those who chose telemedicine for surgical consultations decreased from 72 percent to 33 percent when Covid-related social distancing ended.[98] Elderly patients also find in-person visits easier and more reliable due to telehealth's technological challenges, which can be attributed to insufficient access, low digital literacy, or a combination of both.[96, 115] Many patients will always be more comfortable seeing their doctor in person first and then be fine transitioning into remote care.[116] In the end, the goal should be to make telemedicine an easy option.

It's important to note that the modality of telehealth also makes a huge difference. In one study, 55 percent preferred video communications, and 19 percent preferred phone calls.[92] In certain specialties, including dermatology, patients were satisfied with using asynchronous or chat telehealth options.[117] Regardless of which modality is preferred, patients show a consistent desire to continue to use telemedicine. Even after the pandemic, many agree that they would prefer to have telemedicine remain an option, at least to complement regular healthcare services.[118]

Positive satisfaction and preference are essential for telemedicine to be successful. The main barrier to overcome in the next few years will be ensuring that the public doesn't associate telehealth with its being difficult to use. Recognize what patients like about telehealth, and provide options that reflect their preferences and fit their needs.

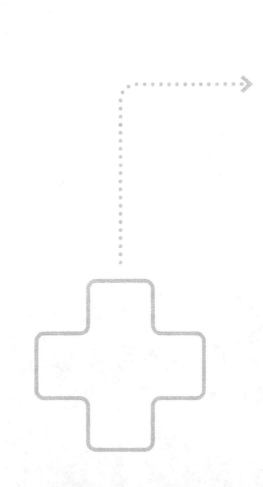

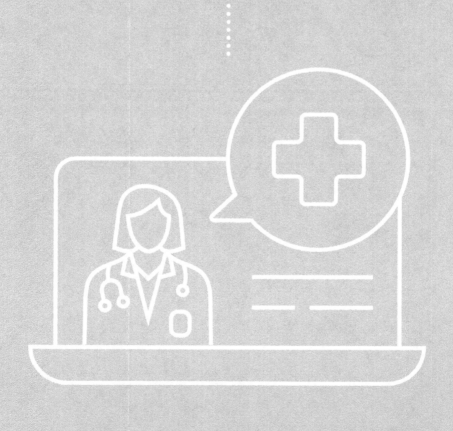

Clinician Success

Aditi U. Joshi

When I started working at Doctor on Demand, telehealth wasn't well known even among clinicians, so I spent a lot of time with colleagues explaining telemedicine. Most of them found it interesting and thought it made sense in theory, but few were willing to *do* it. I suspect that some thought that my focusing on it would tank my career. In the prepandemic years, I had numerous conversations with colleagues about the validity of telehealth. Though most were willing to listen, mostly as a professional courtesy, few had genuine interest.

While Covid rearranged the playing field, it didn't necessarily make telehealth any easier for most clinicians to accept, especially amid so many unanswered questions. In the end, it's important to remember that telehealth doesn't fundamentally change clinical practice; it's simply a different *modality* of delivering care.

In the adoption lifecycle of technology, any successful innovation is carried through its initial stages by innovators and early adopters. It almost always takes time and patience for new things to catch on, and this is particularly true within medicine. Healthcare has a reputation for being difficult and slow to change, but it's not because doctors themselves are necessarily stubborn. It's more accurate to say that few will truly adopt anything without solid data confirming its safety and efficacy. For better or worse, clinicians often end up being gatekeepers simply because making life-or-death decisions regarding a patient's health is not something that anyone is going to take lightly.

Thus, it stands to reason that for telehealth to be successful, the clinical workforce needs to be satisfied with it. If clinicians aren't successful, the adoption and value of telehealth will be limited. Many factors affect the successful adoption and utilization of telehealth by clinicians and organizations: they must consider how to effectively deliver care remotely (chapter 4), it has to be acceptable and satisfying to them (chapter 5), and they must have the full support of their broader organizations (chapter 6).

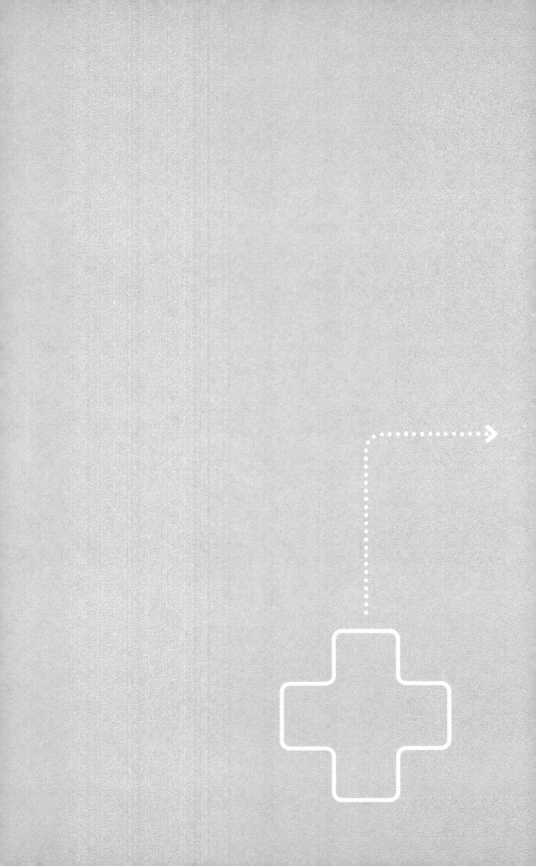

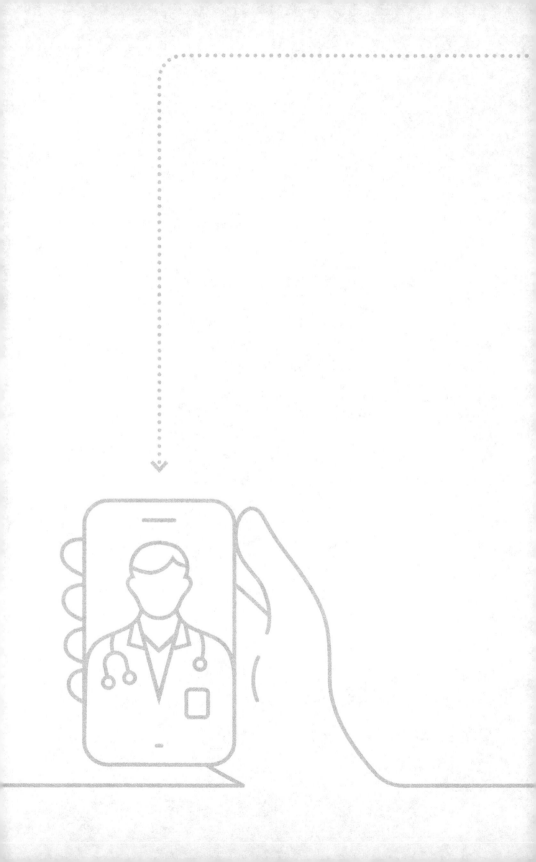

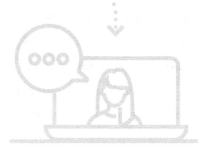

CHAPTER 4

Clinical Impact on Workforce

Healthcare careers have changed enormously in the last few decades. Most newly minted clinicians assume they're about to embark on a long and rewarding journey contributing to society and helping patients. Completing training is a notoriously long and arduous process, and by the time it's over, most are more than ready to get out there and start helping people.

Sadly, it doesn't always pan out that way, and I can say so from experience. After four years as an attending physician in an emergency department, I was already showing signs of severe burnout. More than anything, it was hard to keep up with the sheer volume of patients. The care we were providing didn't always feel safe. Many patients' needs weren't being met, and many couldn't afford their care. Many would or could have been better served elsewhere and ended up in our emergency department only because the broader healthcare system failed to accommodate them. The systemic issues felt endless, and feeling incapable of helping in a real way made it hard to feel good about my vocation. The job I loved gradually became one I dreaded.

Most clinicians enter the field wanting to care for patients but soon they find that doing so is, at best, an uphill battle. There are too many patients and not enough resources to adequately care for them, leading to physicians' burnout and moral injury. As I was contemplating a career change in 2013, I discovered telehealth. I

> **Telehealth added a purpose to my broader medical practice and made me feel like I was making a difference again.**

always had an interest in tech and this was a bridge to continue in the medical profession. Telehealth also gave me room to evaluate and heal from the aspects of my EM practice that had caused my burnout. It also bridged many of the access and care issues that had bothered me. As I continued working in telehealth, I became increasingly committed to using it to improve emergency care. My love of practicing medicine, and specifically emergency medicine, was gradually renewed— something my 2013 self would've never thought possible. Telehealth added a purpose to my broader medical practice and made me feel like I was making a difference again.

Though my story ends positively, the broader clinical workforce is still in dire need of help. The issues I faced were in no way specific to me, and I do not personally know a single clinician that thinks the healthcare system is better now than it was before. With all of this in mind, this chapter will explore how telehealth can, at the very least, improve clinician efficiency and satisfaction.

Efficiency

Care fragmentation, ineffective technology use, inconsistent processes, and convoluted regulatory and reimbursement requirements contribute to a sense of healthcare inefficiency. Efficiency is required in healthcare to make best use of resources and finances and to ensure there is no missed opportunity to care for the largest amount of the population. Particularly for clinicians, it's hard to do your job well if you're unable to be efficient.

Telemedicine can help in a variety of ways, and patients missing appointments is a great place to start. Missed appointments are disruptive, require time-consuming rescheduling and reshuffling, and cause clinics to lose money.[119] Transportation issues are one of the reasons patients miss appointments. Those who rely on public transportation or who do not have access to a vehicle often have the most difficulty, particularly if their clinic or hospital is distant. As a result, many clinics and health systems offer telehealth as a solution. Studies consistently show that telehealth is strongly associated with fewer missed appointments—especially for patients in urban areas who seek mental health services or who have chronic conditions.[120] A study at one clinic demonstrated a telehealth no-show rate of 7.5 percent, compared to a prepandemic in-person no-show rate of 29.8 percent.[121]

Schedule disruptions are the next obvious target. Because clinics run on tight schedules, late patients, longer-than-anticipated appointments, and clinical bureaucracy all have a net negative impact on efficiency. Fortunately, telehealth visits also take less time than in-person ones. One study found that a majority (52.5 percent) of clinicians reported that appointments by telehealth were more efficient than in person.[122] One study found that in-person urgent care visits on average took seventy-one minutes from start to finish, whereas the average telehealth visit took only nine, largely because telehealth required less time for registration and did not entail sitting in a waiting room.[123] Similarly, a study within an emergency department found that the average in-person visit took seventy-eight minutes, whereas virtual visits took merely twelve.[124]

One of the least-loved parts of the patient experience is the waiting room, which has somehow managed to work its way, in digital form, into telehealth visits. In some ways, telehealth waiting rooms are worse than those found in brick-and-mortar offices. They don't always offer the opportunity to ask preappointment questions or to receive notice when the doctor's running late. One surprising study found that clinicians were *less* concerned about inconveniencing patients when they were delayed via telehealth because those patients weren't in a physical waiting room.[125] In response, some telehealth platforms have added the ability to provide wait time updates and/or send messages to patients, improving the experience for waiting patients.

Interestingly, telehealth appointments also tend to run shorter than scheduled. In a study examining visit times in children's hospitals, telehealth visits for behavioral health, physical therapy, and specialty consultations were all shorter than the time originally scheduled.[101] For telehealth schedulers to shorten appointment times, everything must run smoothly—it's critical to note that most telehealth scheduling disruptions are due to technical issues, *not* the need for more clinical time.[126] When clinical schedules are optimized, clinicians can see more patients more effectively, sparing patients long waits. Conversely, when they're not optimized, the entire care process can swiftly break down.

Fortunately, telemedicine scheduling is fairly straightforward, especially when you use the right tools. For telehealth to seamlessly integrate into clinicians' schedules and workflows, clinical staff should be in place to ensure that patients are present and ready—and that the necessary equipment is set up for the attending clinician. Bouncing back and forth between in-person and telehealth appointments can be challenging, and many clinicians, including many of my surgeon colleagues, prefer to block off telehealth-only days, or at least mornings or afternoons.

Telemedicine improves efficiency, for hospitals in particular. Safely freeing up rooms as soon as possible is crucial for patient turnover, and moving admitted patients out of the ER at the right time allows more patients to be seen. One study of hip replacement patients found that using telemedicine led to shorter hospitalization length, a shorter time until the first physical therapy session, and more frequent discharges back home—all with no difference in clinical outcomes or mortality.[127] Incidentally, using telemedicine to screen patients off-hours is also beneficial to emergency departments.[128]

Unnecessary readmissions are another huge area for improvement, partly because they're complicated to address. Patients with chronic conditions in particular are often readmitted for new complaints, often due to comorbidities.[129, 130] Reducing readmissions requires adequate follow-up support, patient education, and discharge planning—all of which can be time consuming and expensive, particularly when done in person. Telemedicine helps with all of the above, and at a lower cost.[131] Studies have shown telemedicine to have the same quality outcomes as in-person follow-up care in heart failure patients. Compared to those who had no follow-up care, both telehealth and in-person patients had *reduced* readmission rates.[60] While studies haven't shown that telemedicine *always* decreases readmission rates, it does typically have the same result as in-person follow up care, and at a lower cost.

Telehealth has also vastly improved "care coordination," which refers to the deliberate organization of patient care activities and general information sharing among all of a patient's care team and care partners. The goal of care collaboration is to ensure that patients receive the right care at the right time, reduce medical error and waste, and generally improve outcomes. Coordinating care across multiple people, particularly in real time, can be challenging to do in person. Doing so requires getting to know the whole patient, a process that involves understanding all the points at which they receive care, assessing the totality of their medical data, and using all of the above to form a cohesive plan. If anything is missing, or if the patient doesn't receive necessary clinical plan updates, inconveniences and delays inevitably follow. The situation is more difficult for medically complex patients, who often need information or interventions immediately.

Telehealth facilitates improved communication and informational sharing between clinicians in a variety of ways, including video visits, asynchronous telehealth, and phone calls. Already, telehealth care coordination programs have been shown to decrease the number of unplanned visits needed for medically complex children,[132] reduce avoidable hospitalizations in diabetics,[133] and lead to better care access for HIV patients.[134]

Clinician Satisfaction

Convenience, satisfaction, and preference in telehealth are almost always discussed from the perspective of the patient, but the clinician perspective can't be overlooked, especially because clinician satisfaction has been deteriorating for years. With many people leaving and fewer going into medicine, the general shortage of physicians between primary care and specialties is projected to be between 54,000 and

140,000 by 2033.[135] A 2022 American Medical Association (AMA) survey showed a 4 percent decrease in physician job satisfaction from 2019 to 2020,[136] and another survey reported a notable increase in "exhaustion and depersonalization" in 2021.[137] It goes without saying that this ongoing exodus of healthcare professionals from the workforce places an ever-increasing burden on those who remain in practice.

There are several clear reasons for low job satisfaction among healthcare providers. They often work long hours in high-pressure environments, frequently without the necessary resources to perform their jobs effectively. Some feel that they do not have enough autonomy or control over their work because of poor management, lack of direction, unclear expectations, and lack of support—all of which leads to frustration, dissatisfaction, lack

> **When done right, telehealth can help clinicians have greater satisfaction in their careers and reduce burnout.**

of motivation, stress, burnout, and worse. The pandemic put additional strain on the healthcare system; as a result, trends have generally continued to worsen.

When done right, telehealth can help clinicians have greater satisfaction in their careers and reduce burnout. Without being tied to a location, telehealth allows clinicians to have more flexibility in designing their work schedules and gives them the freedom to choose between more free time, or seeing more patients in a shorter period of time. Dr. Laura Forsyth lives for half of the year in Turks and Caicos while keeping her full load of psychology patients back in California. Her ability to take an evening walk on the beach immediately following her last appointment has made a huge difference.[c]

With the prepandemic era mostly in the rearview mirror, physicians now have generally positive attitudes toward telehealth. In a review of five studies, clinician satisfaction with telemedicine averaged 78 percent and was above 80 percent in four of the five,[109] and 67 percent of physicians report that they enjoy telehealth video visits.[138] Another survey found that a majority of clinicians (55 percent) reported that telehealth improved their work satisfaction,[139] while some 42 percent preferred using telemedicine over in-person visits when possible.[140] The AMA found that enthusiasm for telehealth has generally increased since 2019 and through 2020. It also found that 80 percent of physicians used telehealth, planned on continuing to do so, and anticipated adding more remote devices and home monitoring to their practices.[141]

Leveraging remote nursing care can decrease the burden on in-person nurses. A friend of mine, Jenna Morgenstern-Gaines, created a virtual care company called PocketRN. Their research suggested that up to 40 percent of inpatient and 90 percent of outpatient nursing could be done remotely. Today, her service is changing the assumption that all inpatient work must be performed in person. Her company's telehealth services include alerts, discharges, and checking on labs. It also provides support for in-person nurses in dispensing medication, completing procedures, and monitoring for signs of worsening conditions from home.

However, satisfaction with telehealth is not unanimously strong among clinicians and generally lags behind patient satisfaction. A study in Korea showed 86 percent of patients were satisfied with tele-

---

c   https://doxy.me/en/resources/podcasts/
    ep-3-telemental-health-from-turks-caicos-with-dr-forsyth/.

medicine compared to only 53 percent of doctors.[142] There are many causes of clinician dissatisfaction with telehealth, but poor audio and video quality rank among the highest. When providers experienced poor audio and video, they were three and half times more likely to be dissatisfied with telehealth.[138]

Similarly, telehealth has a less dramatic effect on a clinician's sense of convenience. One survey found that while 66 percent of patients and clinicians think telehealth is convenient for patients, only 36 percent of clinicians find it convenient for themselves.[143] This is likely because many clinicians still have to travel to a physical office, and telehealth involves an extra step.

The current incarnation of modern telehealth expanded hastily during an international emergency, and more than anything, it was mostly the lack of training that led to poor workflow implementation. Many clinicians had to figure out the telehealth technology with minimal support and then adopted inefficient workflows or usage patterns along the way. Only the largest health systems had staff available to optimize clinical workflows for their clinicians.

Clearly, clinicians' concerns need to be taken seriously; if they are not, many will revert back to in-person visits in spite of what patients clearly prefer. While telehealth utilization has dropped since the pandemic, a broader "return to normal" is a more likely cause than dissatisfaction. As clinics and hospitals reopened and telehealth again became optional, clinicians were able to go back to their old offices, as well as their old habits.

Fortunately, the most effective ways to improve clinician satisfaction with telehealth are mostly clear and simple. Integrating telehealth into the clinical workflows, providing adequate training and support, and keeping reimbursement in place are the best places to start.

BURNOUT

Roughly half of clinicians report experiencing symptoms of burnout, which lead to poor quality of work, increased medical errors, lack of engagement, patient safety issues, poor satisfaction and retention, and early retirement.[144, 145] Burnout within healthcare is usually caused by the obvious stresses of the profession: excessive workloads, high levels of emotional stress, too much time spent on administrative tasks, too little on patient care, lack of autonomy, work-life imbalance, lack of support, and regular exposure to traumatic events. An ugly truth of the medical profession is that mental health issues pervade medicine as much or more than society in general, and the sustained lack of treatment leaves clinicians feeling increasingly alone, angry, sad, or numb.

Burnout increased through the pandemic, when the rate of physicians reporting burnout shot up from 38 percent to 63 percent.[137] It's not just physicians, either; an astonishing 95 percent of nurses reported feeling burnout since the pandemic hit in 2020. The pandemic also worsened attrition, retirement, and dissatisfaction—all of which has led to more and more physicians and nurses leaving the workforce, retiring early, or transitioning into teaching or transitioning from full- to part-time work.[146]

Hybrid telehealth care programs can help avert these issues. One study assessing physician satisfaction with telehealth during Covid found that a total of 76 percent of physicians felt that telemedicine increased their flexibility and control over patient care activities, improved work-life balance for 36 percent, and fewer burnout symptoms for 30 percent. However, telehealth hasn't alleviated everyone's symptoms of burnout, particularly in the case of specialists, surgeons, and those working in surgical subspecialties,[140] but it's certainly helped overall.

Because burnout is multifactorial, it is difficult to fully address. While telehealth can't solve it single-handedly, the easier it is to use and the more it's designed to improve clinician workflows, the more it will increase clinician satisfaction. And telehealth is not a silver bullet. Many aspects of the overall healthcare system need to change, and high-level workflow optimization, training, and team expansion are good places to start.[147] It's important that clinicians are efficient and are satisfied in their work; if not, the healthcare system and the patients within it will suffer. Fortunately, telemedicine has been shown to increase effectiveness and satisfaction among clinicians.

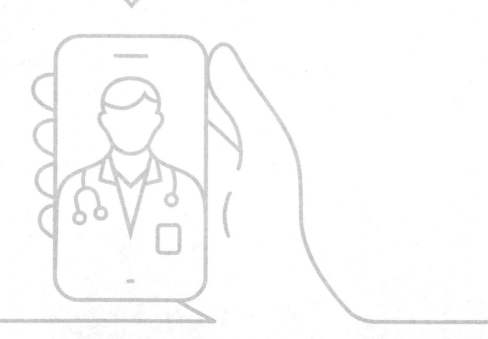

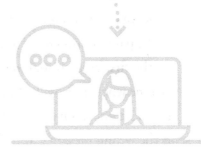

CHAPTER 5

Remote Care Delivery

To be successful with telehealth, it's helpful to remember what *isn't* changing about medicine: delivering quality care will always be the end goal no matter what the modality. However, delivering quality healthcare over telehealth requires its own skill set, and training is both necessary and helpful. Telehealth appointments aren't that different from in-person appointments, but being aware of the subtle nuances that improve the latter will improve remote care delivery. Because telehealth adoption is highly correlated with training and comfort, this chapter covers some of the practical telehealth essentials for clinicians: how you look, how you act, and how you deliver care remotely.[148, 149]

Appearance

Appearance strongly affects patients' perception of care quality, whether in person or via telehealth. The right location and setup can enhance the experience on both ends. Paying attention to these details not only makes you look more professional, but psychologically puts both the patient and clinician in the right mindset.

The first step to looking professional on a telehealth call is to determine where they will take place. Be mindful of your surroundings and avoid unnecessary distractions. Cluttered or dirty backgrounds send the wrong message. You also don't want people walking around nearby where they can overhear your conversations. Set up a designated space where you won't be interrupted. A dedicated space makes it easier to maintain consistency and privacy, though some providers prefer portability, flexibility, and the ability to jump on a telemedicine call wherever they happen to be. In either case, security and privacy are paramount.

Your environment should be as close to a clinical space as possible—professional, clean, quiet, and private. Sitting in front of a simple, clean wall is the easiest way to avoid background distractions. Some providers use a backdrop, an interesting picture, or props for character. Just make sure to avoid reflective backgrounds and mirrors. In the absence of all of the above, most telemedicine software now includes virtual backgrounds that can blur or fully hide your physical background.

Your choice of clothing should be thoughtfully made as well. As a rule, it's generally best to wear clothes that contrast with your background and that reflect your role as a clinician. Many physicians wear white coats during telemedicine visits; if you do, it's best to avoid appearing in front of a solid white background. I myself generally wear scrub tops, just as I would in a hospital.

Your visit also must be private and safe on *both* ends. I've had patients call in from restaurants, while driving, while at work, and other public places. When this happens, I wait for them to go somewhere private, or at least have them pull over into a parking spot.

CAMERAS, MONITORS, AND LIGHTING

Camera placement is another important and often-overlooked consideration within telehealth delivery. The camera should be aligned horizontally and be level with your face so that patients feel that you're making eye-to-eye contact. Your face should appear in the middle of the screen, with enough room to show essential nonverbal communication, gesticulations, and upper body movements. Devices with built-in cameras have the benefit of being placed near the screen, and for those without them, mounting cameras to the top of the relevant computer monitor should do the trick. Pay attention to where the camera is placed relative to where you're looking, especially if you're using dual monitors.

If you're too close to your camera, it can create distorted views of the top of your head or face. I once worked with a doctor who had somehow pointed his camera on the top of his bald head, which his patients understandably found distracting (and slightly amusing). Placing yourself two to three feet away from the camera is ideal because it will give you the appearance of looking at the camera even though you're actually looking at your screen.

Taking care to correctly set up your own monitors will make your calls easier. Doing electronic health record (EHR) documentation while talking to patients on the same screen tends to require bouncing back and forth between the two—and can be distracting for patients. Many clinicians use multiple monitors, split screens, and a telemedicine feature picture-in-picture to do both at the same time. In my tele-triage booth, I set up a large screen for seeing patients on the wall in front of me, a screen in front of me with a camera, and another with an open medical record. With this setup I was able to look forward and have the patient in my eyeline and my body facing the camera, while being able to glance over to see the medical record on another screen. Some clinicians prefer the convenience and portability of using a tablet or separate laptop for the video call, with a separate computer for documentation, which makes charting during virtual visits far more efficient.

Poor lighting is the next most common mistake on telemedicine calls; its consequences create scenarios that range from bad to comical. One doctor I know was appearing on calls surrounded by shadows and darkness to the extent that his patients said he looked like a character in a horror film. A more common mistake is sitting with a window directly in the background, where the backlighting makes the person in frame appear dark by comparison.

Ideally, you should be lit from the front and above. Ring lights are particularly helpful at improving poor lighting and can be placed behind or near the camera. Having a few different, inexpensive, supplemental lights from complementary angles will be the most flattering, if only to reduce deep shadows. Avoid hard light that casts further shadows. Lighting color is measured as temperature—warmer light typically has more yellow color, and cooler light has more white or light-blue tones. The best color temperature for video calls is around 5600K, the same color temperature as daylight.

Webside Manner and Digital Empathy

Once the ideal call environment is set up, the next step is to foster a human connection with patients. Bedside manner—listening skills, effective questions, body language, and the ability to help patients feel at ease—is as relevant to telehealth as it is to in-person appointments. A lot of clinicians learn bedside manner during clinical training, often by simply watching more experienced clinicians, even if they're mostly learning what *not* to do. Good bedside manner does not come naturally to everyone, and most of us have heard stories about or seen doctors who clearly don't have it.

"Webside manner" is the telehealth version of bedside manner, and many clinicians learned during the pandemic that while you *can* establish a human connection remotely, it usually takes some getting used to. While training my older colleagues on webside manner, I let them observe a few appointments before letting them try one themselves. Many thought it seemed simple while observing but quickly realized that it wasn't as easy as it

> **"Webside manner" is the telehealth version of bedside manner.**

looked. It took some practice for many to feel comfortable using body language to engage with patients, but they eventually got the hang of it. Something as simple as hand gestures can foster trust—in fact, three of four patients consider physical gestures important during virtual visits.[92] Clinicians who have good bedside manner usually segue easily into *webside* manner easily, though everyone can practice and improve.

Studies reinforce the importance of building trust with patients, which leads to greater care adherence, collaboration, and fewer allegations of malpractice.[150] Patient-centric communication and rapport building on the part of clinicians are important contributors to telemedicine patient satisfaction.[151] In telehealth, this rapport falls under the umbrella of "digital empathy," which refers to being attentive to patients' emotions, thoughts, and feelings, and having the skill to react to them appropriately when interacting via a computer. In one study, clinicians thought themselves incapable of offering empathy by telehealth and were surprised when their patients found them *more* empathetic in a virtual setting.[152] Ultimately, successful human connection comes down to spending quality time with the patient. When a doctor and patient are not in each other's presence, it's necessary for the doctor to take extra time to truly listen to foster connection and trust.[153] Practice active listening by repeating what your patients have said. Doing so affirms that you've heard and understood them. It often helps to utilize strategic pauses to give patients time to speak, gather their thoughts, or answer questions. Let patients provide their histories without feeling rushed and pay attention to their nonverbal cues.

Virtual History-Taking and Counseling

Dr. Osler repeatedly stressed the importance of taking proper patient histories, a key component of the clinical encounter because they allow us to understand what patients have been through and what's important to them. The goals of taking a patient's history are to further understand a given patient's state of health, determine whether anything within their history relates to their acute complaints, and find a path toward a diagnosis. Fortunately, history taking is not difficult to do during a virtual visit, provided we simply allow patients to speak and listen to what they say. Doing so remotely isn't dissimilar to doing it in person, although we're forced to rely less on immediate physical observation.

It's also required to take the time to deliver news effectively. When discussing concerns and counseling patients, clinicians must ensure that patients know *what* they should do, and *why*. Telehealth is widely used for counseling, and has been successful in VA patients who have multiple sclerosis (MS),[154] need palliative care,[155] and have asked for smoking counseling.[156] It is also used for mental health,[157] addiction care,[158] and even clinician education and training[159]—in other words, anything that would benefit from experts connecting with trainees and patients.

When counseling, clinicians tend to dispense a lot of information, and patients may not always remember all of it, which can lead to improper care at home. Just as in person, it's important to describe things in a way that patients understand. It's not always comfortable for patients to admit they don't understand something, so it's up to clinicians to be proactive. Therapists and counselors in particular often use visual aids, videos, diagrams, and interactive activities to explain difficult concepts and find screen share and whiteboard features within telemedicine software highly useful.

Seeing a patient's immediate home environment via telehealth can also provide valuable insight into their living conditions, lifestyle, and social support network, all of which can aid in making more accurate diagnoses and treatment plans. During virtual visits, I've walked patients through their medication routines, explored their homes in a search for potential allergens, fixed improperly placed splints, demonstrated how to use inhalers, and examined food labels in my patients' fridges, some of which would not be possible during an in-person appointment.

When I started working as a telehealth physician at Doctor on Demand, several patients who had been treated for concussions frequently called in days later with questions about unexpected yet common symptoms they were experiencing while healing. Being able to engage with them made me realize what they really cared about and what remained unclear to them from their discharge instructions. Treating them within their home environments put me in their shoes, helped me better understand what they needed, and made me a better doctor.

Gradually, these realizations led me to counsel even my in-person concussion patients in the emergency department differently. I let them know up front what might or could happen, what was normal, and what was not. These conversations would not have happened without telehealth, and they profoundly changed my in-person emergency medicine practice.

Remote Physical Exams

Of all the questions I've been asked by clinicians about telehealth over the last decade, the most common *by far* relate to conducting virtual physical exams.[125, 160] The concern is understandable and usually comes up when dealing with high-risk high conditions like chest pain, abdominal pain, and shortness of breath.[161] The goal of any physical exam, whether virtual or in person, is *to get information to proceed to the next appropriate step*; there are several ways to accomplish this using telehealth.[162]

Early in their careers clinicians learn that the core goal of the physical exam is identify what's normal and what's not. To do this, clinicians in training are generally shown a full normal exam before learning to identify abnormalities, and then they spend the rest of their careers diagnosing abnormalities. While clinicians learn how to do physical exams in controlled, standardized environments, most patients' home environments are anything but, so the process of doing so remotely requires flexibility and creativity. There are plenty of great resources on how to conduct physical exams via telehealth, and plenty of evidence that low-risk, low-complexity evaluations are safe to do from home.[162–167] Most exams can be completed with the patient alone with good lighting and clear video, but it helps to involve others in their households for certain exam components.

To begin a remote physical exam, start with the *constitutional and vital signs exam*. Assess the patient's general appearance, skin condition, and whether they are speaking clearly, just as you would in person. To obtain vital signs, ask them to count their pulse out loud. Determine their respiratory rate by counting their breaths. If they have medical devices—thermometer, blood pressure cuff, pulse oximeter, and/or scale—you can get the rest of their vital signs through those means. Some patients may have wearable devices that gather this same information; if they do, use them!

The *eye exam* begins with looking at the appearance of the conjunctiva and eyelid to diagnose things like conjunctivitis and stye. Ask the patient to move their eyes to check for extraocular movements. If another person is available, have them use a light to check for accommodation and pupil reactivity. There are a variety of smartphone apps designed for testing visual acuity.

For the *ears, nose, mouth, and throat exam*, start with an external inspection of the ears, nose, and mouth for lesions, masses, and discoloration. Using a good flashlight and the patient's assistance, you can also examine the lips, teeth, gums, external nares, the oropharynx, and the posterior pharynx. For patients with remote otoscopes, you can use that to look for any ear complaints. For people presenting with sore throat, it is possible to take a look at the tonsils with a good light and makeshift tongue depressor.

You can do an overall appearance exam for masses, symmetry, enlargement of the thyroid, and for range of motion in the *neck exam*. With the patient or other family member involved, you can have them palpate the thyroid and the vertebra for pain.

Most parts of the *cardiovascular/pulmonary exam* will require some type of medical device. To start, ask for the pulse, pulse oximetry, and respiratory rate if you haven't already. The patient or family member can palpate the chest to assess for any pain points. You can examine the neck for jugular venous distention and the legs for edema, mottling, or rashes. Next, evaluate the patient for speech, rate of breathing, pursed lips, or any signs of respiratory distress. Heart and lung sounds cannot be evaluated effectively without a digital stethoscope designed to digitally transfer sounds, but some patients, especially those being monitored for chronic heart disease, may have one at home. EKG and heart rhythm monitors, as well as smartphone apps, are all available and can lead to better cardiovascular exams from home.

The *abdominal exam* starts with looking at the abdomen for masses, rashes, scars, distention, and obvious hernias. In pediatrics, you can have the patient jump up and down on one foot, a validated way to determine peritonism. Testing for tenderness will require the presence of someone else because it's difficult to examine oneself. I've demonstrated to available family members how to do this exam, and they've done it under my guidance. A complaint of abdominal pain can be high risk, so it's best to take into account the entire clinical picture; if there is any risk, send the patient in for an in-person evaluation.

Believe it or not, patients have had *genitourinary exams* over telehealth. You can do a visual exam for rashes, appearance, swelling, or any other abnormalities, and patients can send those pictures in advance if they're more comfortable doing so. The patient may be able to aid in the exam themselves under clinician guidance. In general, this is a highly sensitive area. When doing it in person, clinical workflows always recommended chaperones. If you cannot find one for yourself or the patient, it's highly recommended that you suggest an in-person exam.

For the *musculoskeletal exam*, start with general appearance, checking the specific joint being examined for swelling, injuries, rashes, bruising, or any other abnormalities. Under guidance, have the patient move the joint, palpate for pain, and walk, depending on the joint in question. In studies, going through the Ottawa ankle rules (a set of criteria to determine whether ankle injuries require an x-ray) telehealth has been shown to be effective.[168]

If the video quality, lighting, and camera are up to par, a *skin exam* is possible, but dermatologists often request high-resolution images from their patients to improve diagnostics.[169]

Remote *neurological exams* can be tough and should be done only for low-risk cases or when looking for specific abnormalities. Most of the time a neurological exam is used for tele-stroke evaluation, and with another clinician present, but providers can ask patients and family, with guidance, to do a cranial nerve exam and parts of the cerebellar exam. You can evaluate sensory deficits by having the patient use objects such as a pen and paper to test for different sensations. Gross motor abnormalities can also be evaluated by observing gait and movement.

The *psychiatric exam* has been used most often within healthcare that focuses on mental health, an area of medicine that is one of the most frequently used types of telehealth. This exam requires good video, sound, and lighting to really see the patient well and to evaluate their speech patterns and nonverbal cues.

Parts of the exam not listed here may require specialized devices or require in-person examination. For complicated evaluations, suspected worsening conditions, or when the clinician isn't completely sure that the patient can be safely and accurately assessed at home, patients should be referred to a higher level of in-person care.

Even in such cases, patient-run virtual exams still consistently provide clinically valuable information, including the presence of red flags that necessitate a higher level of care.[162] Remember that the point of the telehealth virtual exam is to determine options and next steps, and a remote exam is almost always better than none at all.

Furthermore, involving patients in their own exams tends to improve their health literacy. While working with a patient who presented with abdominal pain, I told them exactly why I was asking what I was asking. By the end of the encounter, they had a clear idea of what signs indicated their condition was worsening, what part of the abdomen had a higher risk of serious disease, and when to either call back or proceed straight to the hospital. I would have never been able to so deeply involve the patient in person.

The remote physical exam will expand in lockstep with technology. A variety of devices such as digital otoscopes, stethoscopes, and pulse oximeters are already improving at-home diagnoses and remote physical exams. In addition, wearable watches and smartphone apps that monitor

> **The remote physical exam will expand in lockstep with technology.**

steps, heart rate, and vitals are steadily generating a vast quantity of clinically valuable health data. Remote devices and home monitoring have created a subset of digital health called "remote patient monitoring," which has already enhanced the virtual care experience and is rapidly becoming the future of healthcare from home.[163]

NONVIDEO VISITS

Telehealth goes well beyond video visits; it also includes care delivered via telephone, chat, and other asynchronous interactions—all of which require additional considerations. Though telephone consults preclude visual examination, clinicians should still follow best practices for listening and speaking. Chat and asynchronous e-visits come in many forms, and are a rapidly growing subset of the healthcare industry.[170] Initial studies have shown that, in thoughtfully designed clinical scenarios, asynchronous telehealth provides the same level of quality as video and in-person visits, and at a lower cost.[170, 171]

Chat telehealth usually entails texting back and forth with a clinician, as well as sending relevant information; sometimes it also involves sending pictures. Success in these types of telehealth generally requires a few things. The first is an easy-to-use chat system. Next, patients need to fully comprehend the questions they're being asked *without* a physician explaining them in real time. Finally, having an agreed-upon time window in which a clinician can reply is of paramount importance. Acute care patients may want a response within an hour, while dermatology patients may be okay waiting twenty-four hours.[117]

There are many ways to improve care using asynchronous telehealth. Some programs have patients fill out a questionnaire before sending it to a clinician, who triages the patients to the next clinical step. Others use algorithms that present options to patients before connecting them to a human clinician when requested or necessary. Often, these types of telehealth visits are used in tandem with video visits, often as a backup, though new and innovative asynchronous-only protocols are being released for specific use cases, including obesity treatment and triage.

To succeed with these systems, it's imperative that clinical workflows are well thought out, and using in-person guidelines is a tried-and-true route to success. Zipnosis, for example, created standardized questionnaires for their patients and clinicians to ensure that evidence-based guidelines for medications were followed, which prevented antibiotic prescription errors, among other things. We'll almost certainly see more of this type of care going forward, so planning for utilizing asynchronous telehealth will help pave the way for your program's success.

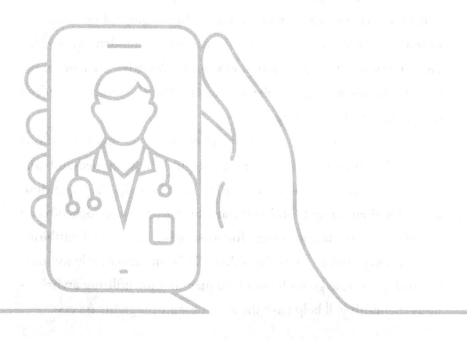

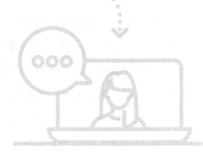

CHAPTER 6

Organizational Success

I n the US if you go into any Level-I trauma center, which is where the worst trauma cases are handled, you might expect to be confronted with a chaotic scene. TV shows tend to depict this environment as noisy and filled with frantic, short-fused clinicians. In the real world, that isn't the case. Within any given emergency department trauma bay, you'll see the emergency medicine doctor at the head and the trauma surgeon at the foot, surrounded by a number of nurses, techs, radiologists, and other relevant doctors. Most rooms are relatively quiet, and people take turns speaking. Everyone knows that the stakes are high, time is short, and action is necessary.

It's a sight to behold, and even after awful injuries or violent attacks, there's an organization and precision that's hard to match. Of course, this level of organization isn't random. Trauma workflows have been designed thoughtfully, and like much within the field of medicine, order flows from protocol. Each person has a specific role, and everyone falls back on their training, and no one person on any team has the skill set to do everything.

The same applies to telemedicine. The cooperation of fully functional teams is necessary to drive change and innovation within all types of organizations. As in all medical systems, telehealth relies on both explicit and implicit hierarchies, so in this chapter, we'll discuss what systems organizations need to have in place to successfully pursue their telehealth strategies, as well as how to support clinician care.

Alignment

Successful telehealth requires a compelling purpose and plan. After all, a vision without a plan is just a fantasy. All stakeholders need to know the plan and have a clear understanding of how to get to the intended destination. Leaving even one group out can stall progress, rack up unnecessary expenses, or even lead to program failure.

The first step toward achieving organizational alignment is to have a clear and high-level understanding of what your organization is trying to accomplish with telemedicine—and why. Your overall purpose for implementing telemedicine may be reducing no-shows, improving patient experience, or increasing patient

> **Successful telehealth requires a compelling purpose and plan.**

satisfaction. In any case, your purpose should be defined and agreed upon via internal discussions at all levels, be aligned with your mission and goals, and be unique to your specific needs. Most of all, be specific. Vague purposes will not get you to your end goal. If you give people ambiguous goals, you'll get ambiguous decisions.

In order to know whether or not your efforts are moving you toward your goals, or not, you need to agree upon measurable outcomes. Many metrics, including no-show rates, are readily available and easy to track, but others may require more coordination, thought, and effort. For example, if your organization wants to improve patient satisfaction, but you don't currently track it, you'll need to implement patient satisfaction surveys over time, ideally before *and* after your telemedicine implementation.

As a telemedicine service matures, it's recommended to have short, medium, and long-term outcomes and goals.[d] It may take several years to reach long-term outcomes, so aim to achieve the short- and medium-term objectives in the interim. An example of a short-term outcome would be getting a specific number of clinicians set up to use telemedicine. Medium-term goals often relate to utilization and usability, which show that your solution is being used and that participants like it. Long-term outcomes could include increasing quality scores, decreasing waiting times, increasing access, lowering no-show rates, and increasing revenue. Having defined outcomes and ensuring you are hitting them at each level will help you succeed and allow you to pivot sooner rather than later when something is not working.

Having a strong leader who supports telehealth can nurture a telehealth program; it certainly helped my team at Jefferson.[172] Our CEO, Steve Klasko, defined our goal as "healthcare with no address" and promptly made telehealth innovation central to Jefferson's broader agenda. Our telehealth program began in 2015 with the overarching goal of shepherding almost all of our departments into doing at least some telehealth visits. Because each specialty has different workflows, we tailored each accordingly. For example, the emergency department did tele-urgent-care-style visits that allowed patients to call in about minor acute care complaints whereas surgeons did postopera-

d   From podcast Season 2, Episode 6: https://doxy.me/en/media/podcasts/
     s2-ep6-improving-access-and-controlling-costs-with-shawn-valenta/

tive virtual visits. As with most innovations, some clinicians took to telehealth more readily than others. Because leadership expected a set number of telehealth visits per department, it went a long way toward increasing engagement, and clinicians found creative ways to leverage remote care throughout a large health system. The expectation was crystal clear: *Jefferson does telehealth*.

Not every system has this type of visionary leader at the helm. More often than not, a specific department or clinic will be the first to try out a telehealth process or program, which can lead to the utilization of numerous platforms within the same health system. To alleviate the inevitable complications that arise, it helps to have a centralized team and a leader who's aware of who's doing what. Over the last few years, health systems have increasingly implemented broad digital platforms or programs, and some have even created centralized digital innovation groups to lead the effort. Involve clinicians, staff, and patients as early as possible so each can provide their own unique perspectives.

The role of *clinical champion* may be the most important of all; people in this role help facilitate implementation and ensure that your telehealth solution meets the needs of clinical users. Chief Medical Officers or Chief Medical Information Officers can also be crucial leaders because they provide input on processes and products and ensure that clinician input is being absorbed and understood. Having this type of clinical leader in place will break down barriers and push telehealth forward faster.

Additionally, there has to be great IT and support staff in place to evaluate, implement, and manage technology, because patients and clinicians will need their help. Bringing in experienced technologists early on can help identify and avoid technical issues before they become bigger problems.

Getting legal and compliance personnel involved early on helped my own team tremendously. When we were thinking of implementing a new tele-triage pilot, they helped us determine what our liability would be if we discharged patients straight from triage, which informed how we created our workflow. In addition to managing risk, there needs to be someone in place who understands liability, can evaluate contracts, and knows what licenses and protections are needed. Laws change constantly, so you'll need competent people around to handle ever-shifting regulations and reimbursement requirements.

Ensure that everyone on that team is seeking the best interest of your patients, clinicians, and organization. Everyone on the team should have the opportunity to attend demos, contribute to the broader effort, provide feedback, voice concerns, propose alternatives, and ask questions. Not all organizations are big enough to have specific departments for all of the above, and in that case, it can be helpful to hire fractional officers or consultants. I can't stress enough how much time and money getting the right information from experts saves. There are simply no shortcuts for getting the right information *before* starting a program.

Finally, you must clearly communicate your aims to everyone involved. Reiterate your purpose, write it down, and reference it often. Your purpose needs to be detailed and informative enough to follow and implement—but flexible enough to incorporate feedback, make improvements, and accommodate your specialist constituents' varied practice patterns.

Understand Your Users

In 1997, when Steve Jobs rejoined Apple, he told his staff, "You've got to start with the customer experience and work backwards for the technology. You can't start with the technology and try to figure out where you're going to try to sell it." This principle applies to how organizations should approach telehealth. Before selecting a telehealth solution, you must first understand what the ideal experience for a patient and clinician would be and design your telemedicine accordingly. Too many healthcare organizations try to fit clinicians and patients to a particular telemedicine process or technology, as opposed to the other way around. If you design the experience around the technology, you give your patients a less-than-optimal user experience, which almost always results in problems and pushback.

> **Telemedicine is impossible without patients and clinicians, so the first and most important thing to understand is *the people using it*.**

Telemedicine is impossible without patients and clinicians, so the first and most important thing to understand is *the people using it*, and they should be the largest influencers in determining how the telehealth solution is set up. Also, every clinic is made up of its own unique blend of patients, so a telehealth solution that works for one clinic may not work for another.

When seeking to understand your patients—their strengths and weaknesses—it's particularly important to assess how technically sophisticated the patients are. They may not know how to download and install software or what a web browser is. Take, for instance, a federally qualified health center that serves underserved patients in the rural South. It selected a telemedicine system that required patients to use their email addresses to login. This didn't seem unreasonable until it discovered, far too late, that many of its patients didn't have email addresses. As a work-around, clinical staff had to spend precious time helping patients set up Gmail accounts, which were then used to create *separate* telehealth software accounts, all to have a simple video call. Had the center understood its patients better, it would have selected different software.

A few years ago, Brandon was a coinvestigator of a research study that assessed the usability of several home-based telemedicine systems.[173] The study found that patients were consistently confused and frustrated by simple things: emails with multiple links, or a requirement to download software to join a call. It was eye-opening to discover the extent to which patients were challenged by standard features. Ever since, he's believed that user experience is the most important consideration when selecting the right technology; in fact, it is *the* key contributor toward satisfaction, acceptability, and the overall success of telemedicine systems.[174, 175]

Thankfully, there are a number of ways to understand your users. First, figure out who your users are by conducting interviews, individually or in groups, with all stakeholders: patients, clinicians, and payers. Surveys will come in handy, and beyond that, there are plenty of readily available data points to be gathered early on. Start by looking at the demographics of your patients as well as data related to the areas you plan to serve. Do your patients take public transport for in-person appointments? How far is your catchment area? How many people in your area have reliable internet access? Do they have computers or smartphones? It also helps to find out from patients about their previous experiences with telehealth. After asking what they liked and didn't like and what could be better, use that to inform your decision.

The next step is to understand as much as possible what the user's journey is to get insight on what they might do, think, and feel at every step of the process. *User journeys* are a great way to do so, and corresponding *journey maps* allow you to visualize the user pathway through a telehealth encounter in detail. Many telemedicine implementations fail simply because they get user workflows wrong. Clinicians already have busy schedules and often run more and more behind as they go from one patient to the next. Expecting a clinician to take additional time to set up a telemedicine system, figure out how to use it, and personally deal with the resulting issues will almost certainly lead to failure. For clinicians, it comes down to this: telehealth workflows must be *as easy or easier* than in-person workflows.

Once you have a telehealth product, allow time for conducting beta testing, processing people's feedback, and making necessary improvements. Even after launching a program, continual improvement is necessary—so don't stop using surveys and interviews after your launch. We used to send out surveys to JeffConnect patients ten days after their visits, which helped us keep track of how we were doing. User testing is a continuous process; user metrics are never static, and your program should recognize that. Ensure you have as many ways as possible to know who is using your product, and how. Once you've gathered information about your users, organize it in a useful, intuitive way.

For patients, in-person visits are often more complicated than showing up for telemedicine appointments. However, if your telemedicine solution requires special hardware to set up, software to download, and/or an account to set up, the resulting burden may offset telehealth's advantages—especially for elderly patients. In sum, vigilantly guard against needless additional steps, requirements, and complexity in general. Ruthlessly evaluate whether each and every step is really and truly worth it. For your telemedicine solution to be successful, it must be *at least* as easy as seeing patients in person, and ideally easier.

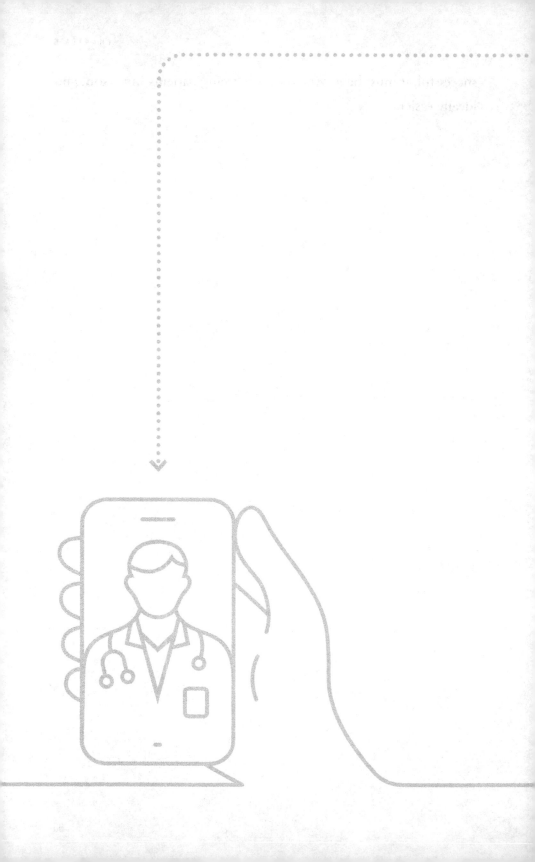

CHAPTER 7

Implementation

I n 2010, a regional trust of the United Kingdom's National Health Service (NHS) spent £3.2 million to purchase two thousand telemedicine units in pursuit of expanding telehealth within its borders. Despite NHS's commitment and an annual operating cost of £600,000, two years later, more than 75 percent of the units sat unused.[177] The first lesson the program administrators learned was that doctors don't want to spend precious time learning and implementing new technology. In response, the NHS paid regional doctors an additional £250 to set up and use telehealth. A program that cost several million to set up and run ended up saving the NHS only £200,000.[178] In a postmortem review, officials discovered three problems: a lack of input and alignment among stakeholders, no implementation plan, and no reason to purchase so much equipment.

As this example shows, a telehealth product and program must be implemented correctly to be successful; a program can often fail because it is not implemented effectively, a mistake that is common enough that a new field of clinical research, *implementation science*

(IS), is thriving. It studies methods and strategies that promote the adoption of evidence-based interventions into regular use in healthcare, including system design, education, feedback loops, and incentives.

> Successful implementation of telehealth goes beyond installing system hardware and software; it also requires effective training and change management.

While there are many barriers to telehealth adoption, technology challenges and resistance to change are among the most prevalent.[174] Successful implementation of telehealth goes beyond installing system hardware and software; it also requires effective training and change management.

Training

Back in 2017, I optimistically assumed that telehealth would be of interest to most clinicians. I created a course while at Jefferson Hospital on how to do a physical exam via telehealth. Part of the course included filming some of my colleagues conducting a physical exam on a medical student and an intern on camera. We used two "patients" to demonstrate how to leverage family members to help with a physical exam. We published the course, made it eligible for continuing medical and nursing education credit, marketed it, and then waited expectantly for it to take the medical community by storm. Imagine our disappointment when fewer than fifty students enrolled.

Fast forward to early 2020 when clinicians were suddenly desperate to learn anything they could about telehealth in response to

Covid. Practically overnight, we had *thousands* of students. Telehealth *seems* like something any reasonably intelligent clinician would be able to figure out independently. After all, aren't we "merely" applying our clinical skills to virtual encounters? The pandemic taught many of us that there are skills and tricks to improve remote care, and many of them are subtle. The most memorable feedback I received came from a doctor who initially told us that the physical exam skills demonstrated in our course video were "obvious" before conceding that he was surprised to find himself *using* those skills on his next telehealth encounter and begrudgingly admitting that the course was helpful.

When fellow clinicians complain to me about their issues with telehealth, my first inclination is to ask whether they were ever adequately trained in virtual care delivery. Most say that they were trained on their telehealth *technology*, but not in the clinical encounter itself. When this is the case, these same clinicians prematurely write off telehealth. In my experience, they have a change of heart once they complete comprehensive telehealth training.

Before the pandemic, large scale telehealth education was nonexistent. Those that did exist were primarily in-person clinical training or distant collaboration. Most were not aimed at large scale education.[179] Adopting telehealth hastily in a national emergency didn't allow for proper training, forcing clinicians to use telehealth platforms that they didn't have sufficient time to learn.[180] Training gaps explain why so many clinicians struggle to connect with patients or fail to conduct physical exams to their satisfaction via telehealth. These two issues led to much of the early dissatisfaction. Education and training improve implementation, and most clinicians agree that training is a key barrier to telehealth adoption.[181] Simply put, the better a clinician understands how to practice telehealth, the more likely they are to use it. Again, most clinicians stand to benefit from more than just technological training. They also need to learn "softer" skills, including how to take virtual histories, conduct physical exams, and know the fundamentals of successful digital interpersonal communication.[182]

While telehealth training is similar across roles, nurse practitioners, physician assistants, medical techs, nurses, clinical telepresenters, pharmacists, and physical and occupational therapists require skills relevant to their clinical role.[183] As a result, professional societies have started creating standard educational models that are specific to various specialties. Initially, most training was nonspecific, but given telehealth's rapid expansion, the industry now recognizes that telehealth education should be *targeted*. As the diversity of telehealth training options has grown, so has a corresponding need for standardized criteria and guidelines. Once standardized, we anticipate that telehealth-centric training will be incorporated into graduate and postgraduate education.

That being said, the ideal telemedicine training program is not specific to any one given medical specialty; it's fundamental skills that can be delivered uniformly across specialties, at different levels and *then* tailored to particular medical disciplines as appropriate.[184] To this end, the American Academy of Medical Colleges created a list of competencies for telehealth education that fall into six domains: patient safety, access and equity, ethical requirements, technology competence, and the ability to connect with patients remotely.[185] These competencies apply to various levels of training: medical students, residents, fellows, new graduates, experienced faculty, and practicing doctors who are leveling up their skills.

Clinicians are busy, so for telehealth training to be successful, it's important to be clear, concise, and in the right format; otherwise, people are likely to abandon the process entirely. A combination of video and text usually works the best, but there are many types of training formats, each with its own strengths and weaknesses.

Online courses are the most accessible because they offer asynchronous learning that can be done at home. These self-guided video tutorials allow providers to set their own pace, and some include tests or certifications of proficiency. While these are efficient for large-scale education, they rarely allow for real-time feedback.

For small and targeted programs, *in-person training* tends to work better. Real-time training with experts can offer a great opportunity to ask questions and dig into topics of interest, but it's not always convenient or accessible to busy clinicians. In-person training is particularly valuable in terms of practicing components of the virtual physical exam with standardized patients, or *simulation training*, similar to how physical exams are taught in medical school.

The pace at which telehealth technology is evolving makes ongoing training and continuing education all the more important. Some telehealth vendors offer formal training programs as part of their service. Many use the "train-the-trainer" approach, which involves a staff member within the organization going through some kind of formal training with a vendor and then training everyone else at their organization. In cases where specialized hardware is used, in-person training is particularly useful, whether it be via a vendor representative traveling to a clinic site, or a healthcare staff member traveling to participate in a training class hosted by a vendor. Within your own organization, it helps to have a dedicated place for educational material, including a simple walk-through of the software you use, or better yet, live or prerecorded demos of your people actually using it.

Managing Change

One of the biggest obstacles to any implementation is resistance to change. When clinicians find a routine that works, most are reluctant to change. At the end of 2019, I was still slogging away, trying to get clinicians to give telehealth a try. When the pandemic hit, traditional barriers were lifted, and for weeks, my phone didn't stop ringing with people asking how to set up telehealth. Regulations were lifted, and telehealth was reimbursed. While the resistance to telehealth adoption has decreased in the interim, resistance still rears its head.

> **Perhaps the most common form is resistance to new and improved telehealth systems.**

Perhaps the most common form is resistance to new and improved telehealth systems. Once people get used to one, it's difficult to get them to switch to another, even if the change in question entails a drastic improvement. As a result, it can take a lot of effort and expense to change from one system to another, especially in larger health systems. To be successful with telemedicine, *expect* resistance to change and adoption, and know the tools and techniques to overcome it successfully.

Because clinicians want the best for their patients, start by telling them why the change will help patients. To help clinicians see this, make the goals and progress of whatever change you're implementing obvious to everyone involved. Measure your performance and results, and directly link them to your stated purpose and goals. For example, if you're implementing telemedicine in a rural practice to reduce drive time for patients, you should be measuring not only the distance patients would have otherwise had to travel but also no-show rates. Keeping a tally of these two items and making the information known to everyone involved will allow them to see the positive impact that their efforts are having with patients. That alone may provide the motivation to keep doing it, even when it means more work for them.

Humans, like all animals, are naturally habitual; we get accustomed to a certain path and tend to stick to it. Clinicians are no different. To make your transition successful, you need to help create new habits with as little turbulence as possible. Again—any new habit should be easier and better than the old habit. In particularly difficult transitions, it can also help to make it hard for clinicians to revert to the old way of doing things, whether by removing access to old systems, withdrawing support, or even making the old workflow more complicated. Of course, this should not be used as the first or only tactic to force change because doing so can come across as controlling, may generate subversive behavior, and/or may make your new program unpopular. Remember that the ultimate goal is to reshape old habits into healthier, more productive ones over the long term.

The best strategy is to understand what motivates clinicians and then use that as positive reinforcement. Some people are motivated by altruism, others by praise and public recognition, and others by financial incentives. A bonus or reward tied to meeting a new telemedicine metric isn't a bad way to encourage a certain behavior. Strategically leveraging motivators can be powerful in overcoming resistance to change, but as in anything else, beware that too much of this can create habits that will vanish once the incentive is removed.

Evaluation

The final step to successful implementation is evaluation. In 2017, Jefferson's emergency department piloted an innovative tele-triage program—one of the first in the country and the first in an academic center. It started as a practical response to a variety of problems. Once we had staffed two emergency departments, we recognized the smaller of the two was failing to meet some of its CMS efficiency metrics.

The first aspect we needed to improve was time-to-provider (TTP)—how quickly patients were being seen by their clinicians. The second metric was our left-without-being-seen (LWBS) rate—when patients leave without seeing a doctor at all. Since we had a telehealth program and trained telehealth doctors, we decided to see whether using remote care would help alleviate the overall problem. We set up a booth explicitly for that purpose, then made sure our telehealth physicians and triage nurses were trained on and familiar with the technology.

The idea was simple: triage nurses saw patients first, took their vital signs and basic info, and then started tele-triage visits with a doctor in the booth. The doctor then saw the patient, asked questions, put in orders, and sent them on their way. Patients proceeded to the ER or its waiting room, started their orders, and then saw an emergency doctor in person. Finally, the doctor reviewed the completed workup, examined the patient, and then discharged or admitted them.

Our hope was that the program would decrease our lagging metrics, get the patient through the ER faster, and generally improve everyone's experience. The results were immediately illuminating. Overnight, even with the program active only seven hours a day, we got our CMS metrics where they needed to be, and patients got workups faster. When we looked closer at other outcomes, we were surprised to find that we weren't getting patients *out* faster. While fewer left without being seen, many left before completing their entire workup, which led to a new designation: "left without treatment complete."[186] This experience reaffirmed the need for real research, as well as the stubborn fact that even things that "make sense" and "should" work may not. Our program was effective for some things, but not for *everything*. We used this data to continue to refine and optimize our program.

Programs that evaluate quality of care and the required steps to improve them fall under the banners of quality assurance and/or performance improvement, both of which help clinicians identify gaps in practice and improve them. To be successful, the goals of these programs and the expectations of the clinicians have to be clear. There are various evaluation methods. Including chart review, evaluating patient complaints, looking at demographics, analyzing various outcome statistics, pulling data from health records, auditing data on telehealth utility, and checking whether patients returned or dropped out of care. Which you use depends on what you're looking for.

Quality assurance programs work and often help both organizations and clinicians meet their goals.[187] After figuring out what's wrong, there has to be a reeducation, a reevaluation, and clearly set guidelines on what needs to be improved. Evaluation is an ongoing process, but it's worth the effort because it reliably improves outcomes and metrics. To prevent oversights, clinical input is essential, including an impartial administrator or at least a genuine desire for group consensus. In the end, the methods employed should find actual gaps in a given program, whether they relate to technology, clinician skill and/or comfort with telehealth, or hitting the program's stated targets.

Creating a quality assurance program for telehealth shouldn't be all that different from those used for in-person care. Unlike in-person care, however, there's a tendency to overfocus on tech failures, user design, and software issues.[188] Be aware of this. Clinical outcomes remain the most useful metric by which to measure and improve your clinical workforce. At a higher level, the main barrier to overcome in coming years will be ensuring that the public doesn't associate telehealth with being difficult to use.

Effective implementation is necessary to avoid failure, and that includes training, change management, and evaluation. To be successful with telemedicine, make sure clinicians receive appropriate training on telehealth, and if necessary, use techniques to get clinicians to change their behavior when resistant, and continually evaluate the impact of your telehealth service to ensure goals and quality objectives are being met.

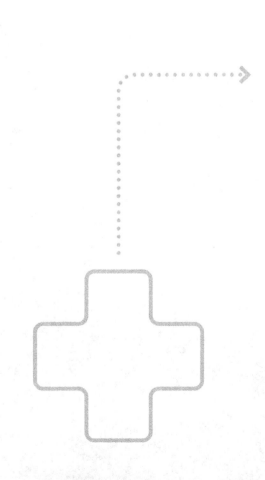

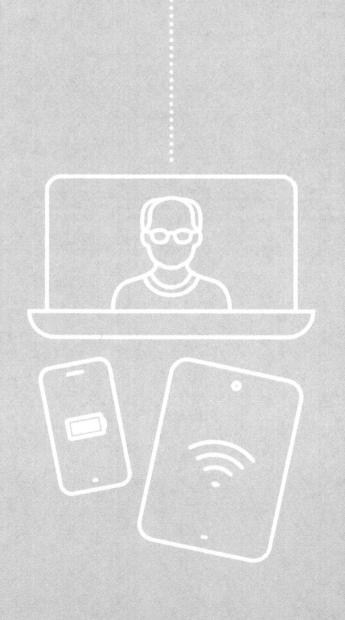

Technology Success

Brandon M. Welch

The Medical University of South Carolina (MUSC) in Charleston, South Carolina, is one of the early pioneers of telehealth; its clinicians started using it in the mid-2000s. After creating a Center for Telehealth, the state legislature began allocating over $100 million to advance telemedicine throughout the state. Since 2013, the center's primary missions have been to administer and distribute telemedicine throughout the state.

For nearly a decade, it has staffed a smart, dedicated, multidisciplinary team of telemedicine experts. The center had the time and resources to vet dozens of telemedicine technologies and work through reimbursement and compliance issues; not surprisingly, it now claims a place at the forefront of telehealth education and training, pumping out academic research on telehealth and regularly presenting at conferences. In 2017, no one was surprised when it was designated by the US Health Resources and Services Administration (HRSA) as a National Telehealth Center of Excellence. For all intents and purposes, the Center for Telehealth was doing everything right.

When Covid hit, anyone would have reasonably expected that its deployment of telemedicine would have been exemplary—and in many cases, it was. The staff quickly built temporary ICUs using telemedicine, placed video endpoints in every hospital room, and implemented large-scale asynchronous and drive-through screenings. At the beginning of the pandemic, the center lived up to its reputation as a telehealth leader.

Then, cracks were exposed. As lockdowns became more widespread, MUSC turned to telemedicine to meet with patients in their homes, which was to some extent new territory for them. They had done small projects with home-based telemedicine using their all-in-one EHR-telehealth functionality. This approach had worked well enough in small-scale controlled settings before Covid, but they hadn't fully vetted and created an ideal set-up for a system-wide rollout.

Once the center began to scale its operation to thousands of users in response to stay-at-home orders, huge problems appeared that couldn't quickly be solved. Its EHR-telehealth functionality lacked basic features, forcing clinicians to follow complex and time-consuming workflows to meet with patients. Even when the system did work, the video service ran on MUSC's self-hosted servers, which quickly reached capacity and caused sessions to freeze, drop, or fail to connect an eye-popping 60–80 percent of the time.[e]

The overall experience was so bad that one MUSC provider described it as "awful" and claimed that "the stars had to align perfectly" just to conduct a simple video call. Soon, clinicians were

---

e   Personal interview with MUSC provider.

preparing to "rise up in protest." Fortunately, clinical groups around campus found alternative telemedicine solutions that worked better and were easier to use.

Despite being a leader in telemedicine in every other way, the center had not provided clinicians and patients the right telehealth technology for clinicians to connect with patients in their home at the time when they needed it most. Sure, Covid was an unprecedented time that no one prepared for, but the core issue remained: *the technology was wrong for clinicians' needs at that time*. Whether during a pandemic or not, to be successful with telehealth, it's essential to select the correct technology for the specific clinical purpose and needs of users.

This section focuses on how to select, set up, and run the right telemedicine technology for your unique situation. Being successful with this sort of technology is so much more than merely picking a product that "does telemedicine." In the next several chapters, we'll discuss how to pick the best technology to get the job done as simply and easily as possible (chapter 8). We'll also dive deeper into how telehealth and internet technologies work, including common challenges that arise in implementation, and how to overcome them (chapter 9). Finally, we'll discuss how to integrate technology into your current health IT infrastructure and workflows (chapter 10).

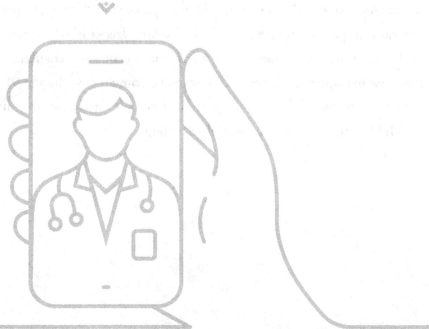

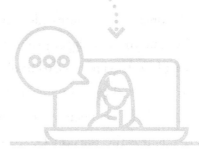

CHAPTER 8

Selecting the Right Technology

"I don't know why they're making us change," a frustrated nurse told me, referring to her organization's decision to move to a new telemedicine system. "The system we've been using works great. The new system they want us to use doesn't notify us when patients have arrived, there are so many steps that it's confusing the patients, and every time we use the new system, we have technical issues. It's horrible!" As a result, she, along with her entire clinic, was flatly refusing to move to a new telemedicine system.

Apparently, the administrators got so excited about a unique feature in their new telemedicine technology that they overlooked how difficult it was for clinicians and patients to have a basic call. The clinicians and nurses were happy with the previous system. The new rollout not only caused clinician frustration, but also resulted in a measurable drop in patient satisfaction scores. Unfortunately, the organization didn't identify these problems until rollout, when it became an even bigger problem to fix. Like many other organizations that have tried to force technological transitions and faced open revolts as a result, they ultimately reverted back to their previous solution.

If you've been in healthcare long enough, you'll probably recognize the tension between what administrators and clinicians want. To navigate this territory, you need to know your purpose, understand your users, define your requirements, and *then* find the right telemedicine solution. There's considerable work to be done *before* finally selecting a vendor, signing contracts, or going live, but getting it done will save untold time and frustration for administrators, clinicians, and patients.

Vendor Selection

Selecting a telemedicine solution is kind of like bringing home a new puppy. The idea of it is fun, but if you don't think through what you will need, aren't prepared, or choose the wrong breed for your family, it will become frustrating. The puppy is fundamentally innocent. *You* need to do *your* homework to make the right choice.

> **Ultimately, telemedicine technology needs to fit *your* workflow, and not the other way around.**

Ultimately, telemedicine technology needs to fit *your* workflow, and not the other way around. While it's possible to build out a telemedicine solution yourself, most organizations don't choose that route. I've gone through the build process firsthand, and it's almost always more expensive, complicated, and time consuming than anticipated. To make matters worse, most healthcare organizations end up with something that isn't as good as envisioned and have to deal with the burdens of maintenance and ongoing support. Because of this, most organizations choose to purchase or license technology from telemedicine vendors.

When you start to explore telehealth solutions, it's imperative to go in with a clear purpose and an understanding of your clinicians' and patients' needs. When evaluating options, have a list of questions prepared, with input from all relevant stakeholders, based on the unique aspects of the care you're delivering. Ensure that you're considering the functions of the platform from patient *and* clinician perspectives. With each telehealth solution, walk through your user profiles, personas, and journey maps to identify user limitations and constraints. Doing so will help you truly understand what you need and will allow them to show you whether their product's a good fit.

GET THE RIGHT PEOPLE INVOLVED

One of the biggest and most consistent problems organizations run into here is simple in premise but has enormous negative downstream consequences: the people making purchasing decisions aren't the ones actually using the technology. Clinicians are often too busy to sit through product demo meetings, and patients are rarely included in the decision-making process whatsoever. As a result, administrators are usually the ones taking the lead on a multistage process of evaluating vendors, sitting through product demos, and asking questions *they* think are important.

When inexperienced administrators are tasked with selecting telemedicine solutions, they naturally focus on features that make *their* lives easier and save *them* time, which often relate to reporting and system management. While they may ask a few questions with the clinician and patient perspectives, they fail to fully take into account the needs, limitations, and experiences of those who use the technology the most.

As a result, patients and clinicians are often left with poorly designed products that they hate using. When clinicians and patients are forced to use telemedicine systems that are not ideal for their needs, they'll waste time calling tech support, troubleshooting, or stumbling through a new interface instead of focusing on patient care. When faced with poorly designed solutions, most will either seek out and use "unapproved" telehealth software, or resist telemedicine altogether.

To be clear, administrator functions should be considered, but only after patient and clinician needs are satisfactorily met. If the patient and clinic experience isn't good, the administrative features won't matter, because no one will want to use the system in the first place. It can't be overstated enough: actively involve clinicians *and* patients in the evaluation and decision process. Throughout the rest of this chapter, we'll describe how this can be accomplished effectively.

KEEP IT SIMPLE

When defining system requirements, keep them as simple as possible. One of the most common mistakes organizations make with telemedicine selection is prioritizing features they *think* they need instead of basic usability. Simplicity is one of the biggest drivers of adoption and utilization—when given two options, users naturally gravitate to the simplest option. Take a step back and determine what's *really* needed. Clearly define and separate the must-have, mission-critical features from the others you

> **When defining system requirements, keep them as simple as possible.**

can live without. Seek a minimum viable product (MVP)—something that gets the core job done as simply as possible.

I learned this lesson when I was tasked with finding a telehealth solution for prenatal care at the University of Utah in 2013. Protocol required that pregnant women measure their weight and blood pressure with medical devices we sent home with them. Initially, we thought we wanted the device data to be sent via the telemedicine platform into the EHR. However, requiring this feature greatly over-complicated the user experience because it required the patient to login with a username and password each time. Moreover, this would have cost tens of thousands of dollars and at least a year to build.

We needed something that was ready to go in a month, so we questioned whether the data *had* to be sent through the telemedicine solution into the EHR. As we explored simpler, less expensive options, we found a way to use the EHR patient portal to allow patients to enter their information manually and send it directly to their clinicians, greatly simplifying the user experience, dramatically reducing costs, streamlining the requirements for the telemedicine app we were building, and getting the product working within a month. Better yet, the hospital IT and compliance departments *preferred* the simpler approach. Had we insisted on our initial requirements, it's unlikely we would have wound up with a telehealth solution at all.

ONE SIZE FITS NONE

When large health systems adopt telemedicine, they usually start off in an organic way with different clinical departments adopting different solutions for different needs. Redundancy, inefficiencies, and lost cost-savings often follow, all of which tend to give administrators heartburn. As a result, many health system administrators seek to consolidate to one telehealth solution for their entire institution because, from their perspective, a single telehealth solution is far easier to manage, track, and control.

However, administrators should avoid the temptation to force everyone to use a single telehealth solution. While doing so might seem easier, trying to meet everyone's needs with one solution is likely to meet no one's. One-size-fits-all telehealth solutions typically add too much functionality for basic needs and not enough functionality for specialized needs—a jack of all trades, master of none. As a result, ER doctors will be frustrated with the lack of features for remote evaluations, whereas mental health counselors will find it too complicated for their patients. Moreover, many telemedicine technologies are designed and optimized for specific clinical situations. If used outside of their ideal use cases, their effectiveness decreases. For example, a telehealth solution that's perfect for tele-ICU is probably overkill for behavioral health visits.

In fact, the bigger and more diverse the organization, the more telemedicine options it should have available. I worked with a telehealth director at a large academic medical center who did this the right way: instead of committing to one telemedicine solution for his entire organization, he opted to have several "approved" solutions available. He likens this to having a "quiver of arrows." When a clinician wanted to use telehealth, he first sought to understand what the clinician needed, then provided them with the best options to match the right product to the right clinical use case.

This approach allows his clinicians to use the telehealth technology that best fits their workflows, instead of the other way around. While managing several telehealth systems can require a bit more administrative work, his clinicians are happier and use telemedicine more. This approach allows for multiple backup telemedicine systems to be available when the preferred system momentarily doesn't work.

While larger and more diverse organizations with multiple use cases will require several telehealth options to be successful, for smaller and more narrowly focused healthcare organizations, a single telehealth solution is more feasible.

FINDING A TECHNOLOGY PARTNER

Dr. Mordechai Raskas, the Chief Medical Information Officer and Director of Telemedicine at PM Pediatrics, has great advice on what he looks for when evaluating telemedicine vendors:

> I actually don't really look at technology very much at all. I prefer to look at the people and the company who are providing the technology, and evaluating whether they're the right *partners*. *Who* I'm working with is far more important than what the technology looks like right now. As long as I know the team working on it is truly going to be a partner, and has the same vision and patient-centered focus, I would far rather choose a technology that's limited in scope, even if it fails to meet every requirement—even if it's 99.9% stable versus 100%.[f]

Dr. Raskas understands something crucial: although there's a wide array of telemedicine platforms, there really isn't going to be much difference. Most vendors use the same underlying technology. As a result, Dr. Raskas prioritizes the nontechnical aspects of the service as *the* deciding factor. He prefers a provider who is adaptive, understands his needs, and will be responsive when there's an emergency.

Focus on vendors that aren't just selling you a product, but who understand what you are trying to do with telemedicine, your unique

---

f   From podcast Season 2, Episode 8: https://doxy.me/en/media/podcasts/
    s2-ep8-delivering-pediatric-urgent-care-with-dr-mordechai-raskas/

challenges, and how their technology can be adapted to best suit your needs. The ideal vendor has staff or consultants who are trained in healthcare and/or have experience running clinics.

Having discussions with a variety of vendors gives you the opportunity to gather information, define your needs, and refine your user journey maps. Telehealth technology experts can provide advice about how best to use their products, point you toward other solutions that may better meet your needs, and show you workflows that go beyond what you thought was possible. As you work with these people, be open to new and better ideas, and be willing to adjust your expectations.

Testing Products

During nuclear disarmament negotiations, Ronald Regan famously used to tell his Soviet counterpart, Mikhail Gorbachev a rhyming phrase in Russian: "*Doveryay, no proveryay.*" In English, that's "Trust, but verify." Every salesperson is going to tell you their telehealth product is easy to use and can do amazing things. The worst course of action is signing on the dotted line without doing due diligence; many who do so find out during implementation that something they were sold isn't actually possible. Anyone involved with selecting health IT products knows how this happens all too often. To avoid this problem, evaluate the system before, during, and after the selection process. There are several steps to follow ahead of your choice. First, learn from others. Talk to colleagues from other organizations about the telehealth solutions they use *without* the vendor present. Long-term users have a valuable perspective, especially in terms of onboarding, maintenance, and dealing with the unexpected. You'll usually get an honest assessment of what works well and what doesn't, what they like, what they don't, and what can be improved.

Ask whether they would make the same choice again and whether what the salesperson says matches what actual users say. If possible, shadow other clinicians and patients using the various products you're considering. Through observation, you may see things that others can't, and what may be a nonissue to someone else may be a huge one to you. Many of your own employees may have used various solutions at previous jobs; talk to them about their experiences, too.

Many vendors publish feedback, as well as surveys, satisfaction scores, and interviews. If they'll share any of this with you, it's worth noting. Many third-party consulting firms and websites conduct telemedicine vendor comparisons. These include KLAS, G2, Gartner, SoftwareAdvice.com, and Capterra, all of which offer detailed reports, product reviews, or customer feedback. Though they're worth looking into, especially early in the process, these should not be your only source because no review site could possibly anticipate all of your organization's particular needs. Talking to real people who have actually used a given product is often the best source of information available.

Next, instead of passively going through months of product demos led by a salesperson, use the system and learn from your own experience. Many telemedicine solutions allow for trial periods. Once you have access to the system, there are several ways to assess the usability of telehealth systems. The easiest is to conduct a *cognitive walk-through*, which involves a small but diverse group of evaluators who use personas and journey maps to step through the user experience and predict behavior in the context of how the product works. A good cognitive walk-through will identify what patients and clinicians are thinking and feeling at each step, as well as any technological limitations and points of confusion or frustration. You're doing more than just evaluating the software; the process involves considering everything else around the persona and their journey to make the telehealth experience work.

For example, if patients are making calls from home, do they have the right devices? Are they up to date? Do they have internet access? Are their connections fast enough? If not, how can they access the technology they need? Does the telemedicine solution require patients to do anything prior to using the software like downloading and installing software, creating a user account, or registering for a patient portal? If so, how hard is that for your patient to accomplish, and how long will these tasks take them? What contingencies are in place for those that need help?

Cognitive walk-throughs are a quick, effective way to identify issues during the exploratory phase, before investing significant resources purchasing and implementing software. But the most comprehensive and informative telehealth assessment out there is to test with *actual* patients and clinicians who actually use the system *in a real setting*. Real-life users are surprisingly unpredictable, and because of this, usability tests are a consistent source of eye-opening insights for system evaluators. Testing things out in real life will show you where users succeed, struggle, and fail—and will allow you to prove and disprove your assumptions.

You can start out user testing with a small number of real patients and clinicians in a controlled setting simply by conducting fake telemedicine sessions. Start by asking users to complete simple tasks like sending a meeting invite or starting and conducting a call. Watch what users do *without* interference or instruction. If they struggle, it's important *not* to give them help or prompts, even if they ask, because it will bias your results. After all, in real life, they won't have you next to them. You will quickly identify certain telemedicine systems that will cause bigger problems for users than others. Five test users is usually enough to identify most major usability problems with a given system.

Once the system passes your user tests, you can expand to more users in a real setting. A pilot test is a great way to work out the kinks and see how a given technology will perform in real life on a larger scale. If you're a large health system, have one clinic, department, or patient population test it out for a few weeks or even month. If you're a small clinic or solo practitioner, try it out for a week or two with several patients. Throughout the pilot, observe several sessions, monitor utilization, and gather feedback from users.

See how your results compare to what you learned from others and the cognitive walk-throughs you conducted. When gathering insights from patients, let them know you are evaluating a system and would like their honest feedback. Most patients have used other telehealth systems or video communication software before, so you can also ask them how your system compares to others they've used.

There are also many standardized usability assessments available to measure system usability, but these tend to be long.[189] Fortunately, short surveys work just as well. In fact, many usability experts are moving toward using the Net Promoter Score (NPS), which is a simple, single question that can capture significant insight. It asks: "On a scale of 1–10, how likely is it that you would recommend [the telemedicine product] to a friend or colleague?" Next, it simply asks, "Why?" When assessed regularly, you can track change over time and compare across other tools and industries. The written feedback from the NPS provides valuable insight as to what people like or don't like about a given telemedicine system.

Selecting the wrong telehealth technology can lead to failure of your telehealth service, but there are many things you can do to ensure you pick the right technology for your needs. To be successful with telemedicine, make sure you have a good relationship with your technology vendor, and when selecting a technology, keep it simple and don't force a telehealth product to do something for which it wasn't intended. Finally, be sure to adequately test the telehealth solution to ensure it meets clinician and patient needs and is easy to use.

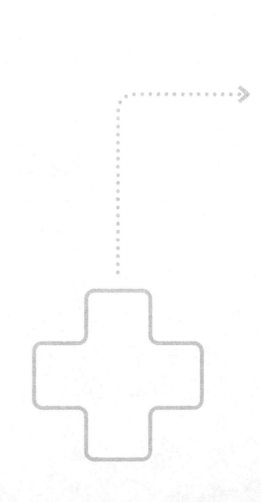

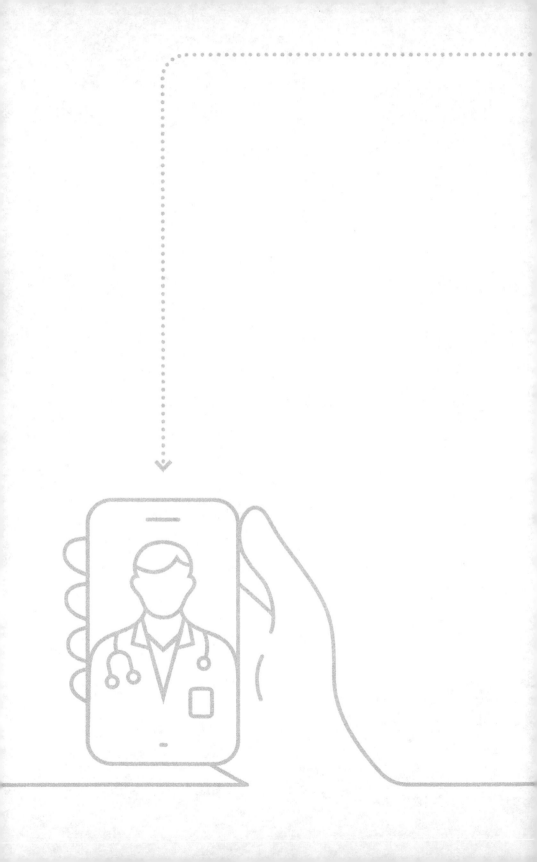

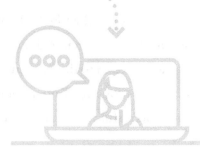

CHAPTER 9

Technology Components

W hen I first created Doxy.me in 2013, it was one of the first telemedicine products to use the WebRTC protocol for video.[190] WebRTC is designed to be built into browsers, so it doesn't require downloading or installing additional software. Users only need a compatible browser like Chrome or Firefox.

When seeking approval from the University of Utah to use it, the telehealth administrator said, "That's going to be a problem because all of the computers in clinic rooms have only Internet Explorer, and the security team wouldn't allow other browsers to be installed." I was quick to point out that they actually had an even bigger problem: none of their clinic room computers had cameras, microphones, or even speakers! The security team didn't allow cameras or microphones on clinic workstations for fear of inadvertent exposure or unauthorized observations of patient interactions by hackers.

As a workaround, we used a separate Chromebook for the telemedicine calls as clinicians continued to use the clinic's computers for documenting in the EHR. This was the easiest solution and was also the set-up clinicians preferred the most because they had full-screen access to the EHR *and* to their patients' video streams. When considering telehealth solutions, it is important to consider all the components required for a successful video call and to ensure they are working correctly.

Endpoint

Every telemedicine call requires at least two endpoints—whether they be telemedicine carts, laptops, computers, tablets, or smartphones. For a time, telemedicine was synonymous with self-contained, dedicated carts that included a camera, speakers, a microphone, peripherals, and other relevant hardware. They were fairly stable because everything was already set up, integrated, and managed—but rolling them from room to room in a clinic requires staff coordination, consistent internet connectivity, and power in each and every room. Their high cost was also prohibitive to all but the largest health systems, limiting the ability to do telemedicine outside of clinics.

> **The industry has moved toward bring-your-own-device (BYOD) software-based telemedicine solutions because they are affordable, easier to use, and more accessible.**

As a result, the industry has moved toward bring-your-own-device (BYOD) software-based telemedicine solutions because they are affordable, easier to use, and more accessible. While software-based telemedicine solutions require little to no hardware installation and use built-in microphones and cameras, they come with their own video quality and connection challenges.

DEVICE

Whether a computer, laptop, smartphone, or old-school telemedicine cart, the device is where visual and auditory information gets captured, processed, and presented to the user. The camera and microphone capture analog video and audio signals that the device converts and compresses (encodes) into digital packets small enough to be transmitted over the internet. The connecting device on the other end of the call then downloads the video and reassembles (decodes) it into the smooth audio and video that we understand as video calls.

Processing (compressing and decompressing) video in real time is computationally intensive and requires significant computer resources. Inadequate or overworked devices are one of the leading reasons for poor video performance. When a device is not powerful enough to keep up with the processing requirements of real-time audio and video, it causes the computer processor units (CPUs) to stop encoding and decoding media frames, causing the video to appear grainy or to freeze.

For a standard 1:1 video call, a minimum of 4GB RAM is typically required for video calls, but 8 GB or more is preferable. For processors, 1GHz is generally the minimum requirement, but a dual core 2Ghz or higher (Intel i5 or higher) is preferable. If your device is causing poor video quality, one short-term solution is to close unused applications or simply restart the device, which often clears up most issues. Of course, the ideal long-term solution is to use newer, more powerful (and expensive) devices, which typically have an overabundance of available processing power. Naturally, a brand-new $2,000 desktop computer will have better video quality than an old $200 laptop.

TELEMEDICINE SOFTWARE

Telehealth software tells the devices in use where to capture video and audio, sends it all to the right place, and displays it properly. At its root, telemedicine software boils down to two types of video technology: application based and web based. Each comes with pros and cons.

Application-based telemedicine software (e.g., Zoom) needs to be downloaded and installed by both participants. The advantage of application-based software is that it has greater control over CPU utilization, media permissions, and hardware—all of which optimize device-related video quality. However, downloading, installing, and updating software can be challenging for some individuals.

Web-based telemedicine software (e.g., Doxy.me) are web applications that run on browsers like Chrome or Safari. Browser-based video is easier for users because it doesn't require download or installation; users can simply give their browsers permission to access the mic and camera when requested. While this type of software is easier to use, they don't have control over device optimization and must rely on the device for video quality.

A few issues may arise with both types of software. While vendors can control the software, they don't control the hardware, operating systems, or browsers that their software runs on. Without this control, updates to operating systems and browsers can cause bugs or problems. For example, Apple is notorious for making changes to their iPhone operating system that cause audio issues within video software.

Out-of-date software and browser versions can also cause issues. Software-based telemedicine applications should notify users when they need to be updated because failure to do so may result in problems. Similarly, most modern browsers automatically stay up to date when they restart. However, if the user hasn't restarted their browser or computer in several weeks or months, they could be using an out-of-date version.

Third-party software is also known to cause issues with telemedicine services. This most often occurs when the service attempts to gain access to the microphone, camera, or speakers, only to be blocked by another video application. Similarly, ad blockers and antivirus software can inadvertently block access to cameras, microphones, or other critical components needed to run telemedicine applications on a device. Configuring the software to allow access to the telemedicine software, or temporarily disabling the service at the time of the call, usually mitigates these issues.

Developing software is a complicated process, particularly when there are many people working on the same codebase at the same time. Human error is a normal part of software development. Most of these mistakes are caught during code review and quality assurance testing, but bugs inevitably get through. Most bugs are unseen or benign, but those that aren't can be disruptive to users. Responsible software companies have a formal process to catch, document, track, and fix bugs to reduce the negative impact on users. If you suspect a bug, alert the software vendor.

CAMERA

Cameras play a big role in video quality. One of my most eye-opening experiences in relation to this happened in 2020, after I'd already been conducting video calls for nearly a decade. One day, I joined a call with an individual whose video quality was better than anything I'd ever seen. His face was crystal clear, the lighting was perfect, and the background was even slightly blurred *without* using the blur feature in the software. We were using the same video software I'd always used. What was the difference?

At the end of our call, I couldn't help asking how he did it. He laughed, said he was a bit of a photophile, and sheepishly admitted he spent way too much time and money perfecting his camera setup at the start of the pandemic. He explained how he converted a $2,000 professional photography camera into a webcam, manually adjusted the camera to focus on his face, and calibrated the ideal exposure and lighting, which created a crystal-clear image with slightly blurred background. I was surprised by how much of an impact the camera made on the perceived quality of the video call.

When placed side by side, it's easy to see the difference between expensive cameras versus cheap webcams. Fortunately, you don't have to go out and buy an expensive professional camera to achieve high video quality. Many cameras provide suitable quality for a few hundred dollars. Also, laptops and mobile devices have cameras built in, and even these are noticeably different; generally, more expensive devices will have higher-quality cameras.

Cameras can be a source of error, the most common of which usually relates to access permissions. Any video software must request user permission to use a device's camera, but sometimes users inadvertently deny access. If this happens, restarting the software to grant permission is necessary. Similarly, if multiple video applications are accessing the same camera at the same time, it can create conflicts; closing the other applications or restarting the device will resolve the issue.

If multiple cameras are connected to a device, sometimes the wrong camera may be selected. Telehealth software usually has settings that allow the user to select the correct camera. Finally, cameras sometimes simply fail to start. If this happens, restarting the device or using a new camera should remedy the problem. Sometimes the camera can appear to be off if something is blocking the camera, like a privacy cover.

Clinicians occasionally ask about PTZ (pan, tilt, zoom) cameras, which give clinicians greater control over what they see on the patient side. However, this requires camera controls within the software and a special, expensive type of camera on the patient end. As a result, PTZ cameras are generally used only in clinic-to-clinic telemedicine carts.

SOUND

Audio issues are also one of the most common problems on telehealth calls. Typically, one participant is simply unable to hear or be heard by the other participant. Like cameras, users need to ensure the correct speakers are selected, on, and turned up. Misselected speakers are one of the most common sound-related issues on telehealth calls. Sometimes it's simply more prudent to use headphones, both for privacy and noise reduction. While Bluetooth headphones (e.g., AirPods) are becoming increasingly popular, they too are known for connection issues.

Just as with the camera, the user must grant permission for the telehealth software to access their microphones. Some devices have multiple microphones, so it's important to be mindful of which microphone is selected. Some microphones have manual mute buttons, so if yours does, ensure you know where it is and that it's off! Sometimes, improperly configured microphones can create a distracting feedback loop; using headphones usually solves this problem. It is good practice to simply test the audio before each telehealth call.

Some microphones are not as good at distinguishing human voice from background noise, and excess noise distracts participants. Other microphones can be finicky and need proper placement to pick up sound clearly. Like cameras, built-in speakers and microphones are usually good enough for the purposes of telehealth, but better-quality microphones can improve both the audio quality and the experience of patients and clinicians.

Internet Technology

It's amazing to think about: today, we're able to sit on one side of the globe and instantaneously speak with someone on the other side of the globe in real time almost as if we were sharing the same space. Information travels thousands of miles in the blink of an eye. Our ancestors, many of whom spent months traversing oceans, would be astonished by it—yet now it's something many of us take for granted. Despite this miracle of technology, poor video and audio quality and dropped connections are a major source of frustration for telehealth users.[175]

For video communication over the internet to occur, everything must work together. The path of audio and video data from one location to another on a telemedicine call over the internet is fairly straightforward; the internet is made up of many devices (endpoints) linked together in a network that can transfer data between each other. A single computer connects to the internet through routers and modems to internet service providers (ISPs), and telehealth services facilitate a connection between the desired participants.

Since audio and video are simultaneously being sent (uploaded) and received (downloaded), providing a smooth video experience requires significant bandwidth. Bandwidth is the total amount of data, measured in "bits per second," that can be transferred on the specific network in a given timeframe. Bandwidth provides the *potential* for high speed, but if there's a lot of data traffic, that data will be forced to move more slowly. It is comparable to the lanes on a highway: the more cars taking up lanes on the highway, the slower the cars can travel. Overall bandwidth is influenced by many factors, including your ISP, Wi-Fi, and device.

If there's no disturbance on the network, and internet connections on all sides are stable and strong, audio and video data packets will flow without issue, and the video call will work seamlessly. On the other hand, if there's a bandwidth failure, limitation, or slowness *in any step along the path*, audio or video packets will be lost, resulting in choppy video and audio, freezing, degraded video quality, and dropped calls. No matter how good your device or telemedicine service is, if the internet connection is poor, it will lead to a low-quality telemedicine call.

One of the biggest mistakes clinicians make when troubleshooting video calls is the failure to consider *both* sides of the call. It sounds so simple, but *both* participants need to have a good internet connection and a sufficiently powerful device to have a good video call. I've talked to so many clinicians who complain about call choppiness despite brand-new computers and fast internet. Many don't realize that it doesn't matter how good a computer and internet connection *you* have. If your patient's using a ten-year-old computer with poor Wi-Fi, the call quality will be poor. In fact, most issues actually tend to occur on the patient side, especially if they're at home. A 2021 Pew Research study found that 30 percent of adults often or sometimes experience problems connecting to the internet at home, and 9 percent say such problems happen often.[191]

> **One of the biggest mistakes clinicians make when troubleshooting video calls is the failure to consider *both* sides of the call.**

WI-FI

Wi-Fi is one of the biggest sources of internet-related failure on telemedicine calls. Most people place their Wi-Fi routers in a dark, obscure corner of their home or office, often in places where they won't be having calls. Unfortunately, a Wi-Fi signal degrades as it travels over distance, passes through walls, or collides with the signals of other electronic devices in the vicinity. A poor Wi-Fi signal isn't noticeable when browsing the internet or sending chat messages because the delays are so short, but that same short delay during a real-time video call is disruptive.

Wi-Fi also is also greatly affected by concurrent usage. There is only so much bandwidth a Wi-Fi router can support. If there are multiple devices streaming Netflix, gaming, and downloading music, there is only so much bandwidth left for video calls. Clinic and public Wi-Fi networks often have many concurrent users eating up bandwidth, and together, this traffic congestion on top of a poor Wi-Fi signal will cause data packets from the telemedicine call to drop, reducing call quality.

If you or your participant are experiencing poor call quality, the first step is to determine if it's related to Wi-Fi and whether it can be fixed. Most devices have an indicator that shows the Wi-Fi strength. If you have a poor signal, simply move closer to the Wi-Fi router, upgrade to a new one, or install router extenders, repeaters, and/or mesh networks to boost signal strength, quality, and speed. To avoid these issues from happening during a call, it is best to check signal strength and conduct speed tests before the call to ensure that Wi-Fi is strong enough once the call starts.

Many forget that the best way to avoid Wi-Fi issues is *to not use Wi-Fi*. Wired connections are often ten times faster than Wi-Fi and mitigate issues caused by interference, distance, and concurrent usage.[192] Although most desktop computers today still have ethernet ports, many laptops today do not, in which case people should use an inexpensive USB ethernet adapter.

Finally, many networks may also include firewalls to filter out unwanted or malicious internet traffic. Though they're meant to protect networks from harm, firewalls themselves can also cause connectivity issues. If their security rules are set up to be restrictive, they can often unintentionally block telehealth applications. If this happens, the telemedicine app won't appear to connect the patient and provider, and it might not be entirely clear *why* the call is failing to connect. While firewalls are used everywhere, those at hospitals are often stricter than home networks. Because of this, a network administrator needs to add an exception to the firewall's rules to allow the telehealth app to work correctly.

INTERNET SERVICE PROVIDERS

Before you get excited about expanding telehealth access, the internet has to be available and work. Telehealth technologies rely on the public internet to transfer data, and access to that comes from several types of internet service providers (ISPs), each with its own strengths and limitations.

Wired internet, including cable, fiber, and DSL, are the most common forms of high-speed internet. Cable internet uses existing cable TV lines to connect to the internet via coaxial cables. It's fast, reliable, and the most widely used way to connect to the internet today, but it is limited to metropolitan areas with populations that can justify and support the necessary infrastructure. Fiber internet, which uses fiber-optic cables to connect to the internet, is newer, faster, and promises speeds much faster than cable but is expensive to roll out. DSL (digital subscriber line) uses telephone lines to deliver internet to rural areas but is limited by slower speeds.

Those without wired internet access often use satellite ISPs, like HughesNet or Starlink. Satellite internet companies are able to deliver high speed internet to rural locations, but they're expensive and can have their own connection issues. "Dial-up" internet, which is also delivered through phone lines, like AOL, is too slow for real-time video and has generally fallen out of use.

Mobile devices now account for the majority of web traffic.[193] When not using Wi-Fi, smartphones connect to the internet via cell towers, and network technology (3G, 4G, LTE, 5G) is continually expanding to support more bandwidth, speed, and concurrent usage. However, as anyone with a smartphone knows, not all places have access to strong enough cell tower signals to provide a reliable internet connection.

Furthermore, even though a user may have a good cellular signal, if there are a lot of people using the same cellular towers at the same time, the internet speed can dramatically slow down. Natural disasters can also cut out power to cell towers, preventing any connectivity. If your smartphone connection is slow due to congestion, try connecting to a Wi-Fi network that uses a hard-wired ISP. Conversely, if you suspect an issue stems from your Wi-Fi or wired ISP, you can switch to a cellular connection to assess if its connection is better.

ISPs themselves can also sometimes be the source of the problem. ISPs and cellular providers reserve the right to control how their networks are being used.[194] For instance, as the pandemic lockdowns caused more people to stay home, people increasingly relied on the internet for both work and entertainment. With more and more people online, wired ISPs saw a significant increase in internet traffic, and the resulting congestion caused slower internet speeds by as much as 38 percent.[195] Additionally, it's common for ISPs to slow down their services for users with cheaper internet plans and prioritize users who pay more. If your internet service is throttled, it may cause video quality issues. If you suspect that your connectivity issues stem from your ISP, contact them.

Support

No technology always works as intended. When call quality is poor, a user interface isn't intuitive, or something breaks, users need to receive the right support at the right time. Effective technical support is essential for telemedicine to be successful. If support isn't in place, both clinicians and patients will struggle.

For better or worse, the first line of technical support is often the clinician. One clinician remarked that once he "learned the tricks" to a good telemedicine call, his issues declined dramatically. He habitually had his patients restart their devices, made sure they closed bandwidth-hungry applications, and asked them not to use Bluetooth microphones.

> **Effective technical support is essential for telemedicine to be successful.**

Basic training is consistently beneficial. When clinicians are able to identify the potential source of tech-related problems, most issues can be resolved within a minute. Waiting on support staff to fix the problem usually takes more time and effort, even for minor issues. Interestingly, patients report being more engaged and satisfied when *clinicians* are able to provide basic support.[175]

That being said, clinicians can't afford to take too much time from seeing patients to deal with technology issues. At Jefferson, Aditi and her team tried to resolve problems *before* the call by making sure patients could log in to their visits before they started, sometimes even a day or two in advance. In this case, hospital staff end up providing a lot of technical support, so they too should have a basic understanding of how to resolve technical issues.

For more complicated situations, you will need a team of IT support professionals. Some telemedicine technologies include support as part of their offering, and others leave support to the healthcare organization. The pros and cons to each approach follow. *Vendor-based support* is provided directly to clinicians, and sometimes even to patients. The advantage of this type of support is that representatives tend to be well trained on their products and can detect issues and provide a resolution quickly, often simply because they've seen the same problem many times before. Vendor support agents can detect patterns of issues trending among users and even preemptively notify them before they become a real problem. However, they do not have direct access to the devices or local networks used by participants, so it may be harder to directly fix a device or network issue on their own.

Many large health systems prefer to be the first line of telemedicine support and thus rely on *in-house support* from their own IT support teams. In-house support teams have a better understanding and more control over the devices and local networks, but these teams can be expensive, especially if used across multiple locations or during nonpeak hours. Given its high cost, dedicated full-time internal support is generally practical only for large health systems with correspondingly large budgets.

Regardless of *who* provides the support, there are many ways it can be delivered. Ideally, a telemedicine product should self-detect that an issue is happening and provide an automated, in-the-moment notification with steps to overcome the issue. Semiautomated chatbots can also be useful to provide first-level support and guide users to the right solution quickly. However, if they're not designed thoughtfully enough to get users to the right solutions quickly, they'll make the user experience even more frustrating and time consuming. Passive self-service solutions, such as help pages, user manuals, YouTube videos, or a good old-fashioned Google search can help users get solutions to their problems but require more effort on their part.

Fundamentally, users are looking for resolutions to their issue quickly, particularly if the issue is happening *during* a call. Many prefer talking to a human right away. Human support can be provided in real time through chat, phone, and video—or asynchronously through email or a ticketing system, which may take hours or days. Humans are a limited resource, so there are often queues to speak to agents, particularly during busy times; it's wise to pay close attention to resolution times in service-level agreements.

Finally: things break. It's not an issue of if, but when. Outages can be especially frustrating for users, so when one happens, communication is paramount. Users should know the system status and an estimate for when regular service will resume, often through a temporary landing page, banner, or alert. Some telehealth services send out emails or use social media to keep their users in the loop. Responsiveness to problems defines how resilient and responsive an organization is.

Technology is one of the biggest sources of failure for telehealth, and technology failure consistently leads to lower satisfaction among patients and clinicians. There are many components that must work together to make a successful telehealth call, and once one fails, the telehealth encounter itself stands to fail. To be successful with telemedicine, ensure that both clinicians and patients have a good computer or smartphone as well as fast, unobstructed internet connections. Also be sure that cameras, microphones, speakers, and peripherals are set up and functioning properly. Learn and understand the most common contributors to poor call quality and how to circumvent them, whether on your own or with an appropriate support team.

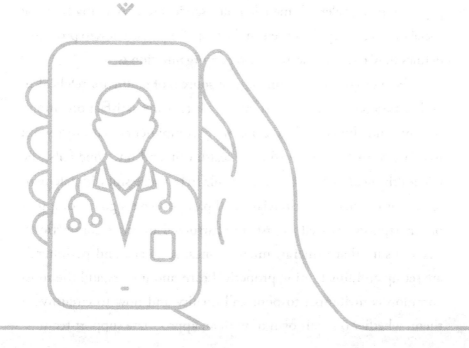

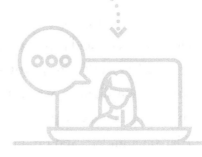

CHAPTER 10

EHR Integration

ompared to other industries, healthcare has always been infamously slow to adopt technology. While industries like air transit and banking embraced change and made new solutions widely available, healthcare continued to lag behind in terms of technology adoption. Up into the early 2010s, most healthcare clinicians were still using paper charts to document.

It's taken two worldwide catastrophes to get to where we are today. First, the economic meltdown of 2008 led to the American Recovery and Reinvestment Act (ARRA) in 2009, which provided $47 billion in stimulus spending for healthcare organizations to adopt EHRs, with corresponding penalties if they didn't.

The second, of course, was the Covid pandemic, which forced the widespread adoption of telemedicine. Without these two seminal events, health IT would probably still lag a decade behind. Even now, digital integration in healthcare still hasn't reached its full potential and may not for years to come. With that said, telemedicine is a digital tool, so we can't talk about telemedicine without discussing other electronic tools and applications, and how they interact.

Today, EHRs document and store individual patient medical information digitally, which is necessary for billing and reimbursement, and track care provided over time and by multiple clinicians. Alerts, reminders, and prompts within EHRs help to ensure patient safety and improve outcomes. E-prescribing and electronic ordering streamlines the communication for ancillary services. Some EHRs also function as practice management systems, which help make administrative and office work, such as scheduling, easier for clinic staff.

Most EHRs also have portals that allow patients to view health information like discharge summaries, prescriptions, immunizations, and lab results. Many also allow patients to message the clinic, request prescription refills, schedule appointments, make payments, view education materials, and fill forms or assessments. At a broader level, EHRs also make public health reporting, population health, and clinical research more efficient.

With a wide variety of uses and benefits to healthcare, it's not surprising the US government mandated the adoption and use of EHRs in 2009. In the subsequent decade, EHR adoption in healthcare rose from less than half to over 90 percent today.[196] EHRs are now a mainstay in clinical practice, and for better or worse, they facilitate most clinical actions and need to be factored into any telehealth decision.

The EHR Paradox

Health IT software is created to serve various needs. Historically, these applications were usually created to solve a single problem, such as patient scheduling or electronic prescribing. As a result, clinics would have to piece together various health IT software applications, sometimes with overlapping functionality, to accomplish a full suite of clinical tasks. To make these disparate health IT systems work together, system integration and interoperability became a major function of the health IT industry. Over the years, many of these health IT systems expanded their functionality beyond their initial scope and merged with other applications to create all-in-one EHRs. Today, EHRs typically provide a digital health record, practice management, e-prescribing, patient portals, and even telemedicine functionality together.

Many healthcare organizations are drawn to all-in-one EHR applications; the management of one application is often easier than several and avoids the need for system integration. While this approach is appealing to administrators, again, these all-in-one EHRs tend to be jacks of all trades and masters of none. Though they may allegedly do "everything," they're rarely best in class at any one feature. As a result, EHRs are a major source of frustration for clinicians.[197] The most common complaints are that they're cumbersome to use, poorly designed, and hinder clinical practice by not accommodating clinical workflows.

> All-in-one EHRs tend to be jacks of all trades and masters of none.

In fact, many EHRs were originally designed for back office administration, *not* clinician workflows. Since reimbursement has the clearest path to value for most healthcare organizations, many EHRs are optimized for practice management and billing. In fact, clinical documentation didn't really become a financial motivator of EHRs until the ARRA was passed in 2009. Today, many clinical workflows are still designed first and foremost to ensure proper documentation for billing.

Understandably, there's tension between what administrators want and what clinicians want from an EHR. Clinicians want something easy to use so they can focus on patient care, and administrators don't want to manage multiple systems. The resulting solution is often a hybrid; using a single EHR for most things and then filling the gaps with third-party applications.[198]

This same dynamic exists with telemedicine in EHRs, which were not originally built with telemedicine in mind. Telehealth isn't the core business of EHRs, so their telemedicine features tend to be pretty basic: simple one-to-one video calls that require prior scheduling, limited in-call features, and rigid workflows. Unsurprisingly, this situation usually leads to poor satisfaction ratings. As a result, over 73 percent of physicians do not use built-in EHR telemedicine capabilities and prefer to rely on third-party telemedicine products for their needs.[199] In response, some third-party telemedicine software has also added basic practice management and patient record capabilities.

Workflow Integration

As telehealth becomes a mainstay of clinical practice and workflows, the question of how to integrate third-party telemedicine apps and EHRs comes up often. Even with a PhD in biomedical informatics, I find it to be one of the most perplexing questions, partly because integration and interoperability tend to mean different things to different people.

Once, an administrator asked whether Doxy.me integrated with his EHR. In response, first I asked him what he was trying to accomplish. He told me, "Our clinicians prefer a seamless experience between the EHR and their telemedicine software. They want to click a button within the EHR that opens up their video call and don't like bouncing back and forth between the EHR and the telemedicine app *during* video visits. We also don't want them to have to remember a separate login from their EHR and the telemedicine software—they have a hard enough time remembering their EHR login as it is!"

This administrator was essentially asking for *workflow* integration. Fortunately, workflow integrations are relatively easy and readily available and don't require extensive and time-consuming technical work. First, I suggested that he configure a button or link *within his EHR* to open Doxy.me, and to use single sign on (SSO) for login. Most large health systems already use SSO, which allows users to log in once with a single ID to access multiple software systems everywhere else. It's fairly standard for EHR and telemedicine software to use SSO, and his organization was already using it.

I also told him that built-in video within the EHR interface is not an ideal user experience for the clinician. I suggested that his clinicians use split-screen or dual monitors, where they have the EHR on their left monitor and the video on the right.[g] Alternatively, his clinicians could also use the picture-in-picture feature, which allows the video of the patient to hover in the foreground over the EHR. None of this required any real technical integration between two systems; the capabilities were all readily available. Once he understood this, he realized that he could accomplish everything he wanted without further "integration" and has been happily using it since.

Similarly, keeping patient workflow as simple as possible increases the likelihood of success. An essential element is sending patients appointment reminders. When invites are sent to the patient from the EHR, they should include all the information necessary to join the

---

g   See chapter 5.

call: date, time, location, and a link to the call. If the telehealth link is static, generic, and unchanging, then no integration is necessary; simply adding the link URL in the clinic location field is enough for integration. However, if the room link is dynamic—meaning it is unique and changes for every meeting—then a "tighter" integration with the telehealth app may be necessary. Alternatively, some organizations prefer to use the EHR patient portal as a way for patients to access telehealth calls; this can ensure that the right patient is in the right place and facilitates the sending and receiving of information.

A word of caution with patient portals: requiring patients to set them up often adds an unnecessary barrier. One large hospital I worked with required patients to log in to their patient portal to join a telemedicine appointment before it realized that less than 25 percent of their patients were registered for the patient portal. To make matters far worse, the hospital required patients to come in person to the hospital to receive a unique sign-up code to register for the patient portal. When Covid hit, lockdowns prevented patients from coming into the hospital to register, so the hospital had to abandon the EHR-integrated telehealth solution altogether in favor of a stand-alone telemedicine solution that did not require on-site registration.

Data Integration

Data integration, or the ability to send and receive data between systems, is the most challenging type of EHR integration, and many want to pull patient data from the EHR to use within their telehealth software. Because patient data privacy is an important factor, *reading* patient information from an EHR typically involves the health organization giving an approved telemedicine app API access with read permissions, as well as a way to link an identified patient in the telemedicine app back to the same patient in the EHR. This complex set of requirements is generally why some telemedicine apps require patient emails, birthdates, or other identifying information during the sign-in process. If patient data—from intake forms, clinical notes, transcriptions, images, recordings, or vitals from medical devices—are collected in the telemedicine software, sending that information to the EHR will reduce the need for duplicate data entry and inconsistencies between systems.

Writing information to the EHR is more difficult than reading. Fundamentally, EHRs are responsible for data integrity, and they don't like the idea of external apps writing patient information to their systems. As a result, they place stringent control over the data they store. Some EHRs restrict where external patient information can be saved, and in what format. Moreover, many EHRs require providers to review and approve data before it can be stored in the patient record.

Additionally, there are *hundreds* of EHR systems, all with their own interfaces and data structures, most of which require custom integration. To overcome this issue, since the early 2010s the US government has been mandating that EHRs use interoperability standards to promote health information exchange. Health data interoperability standards, such as HL7 FHIR, make it easier for disparate health IT systems to communicate using a common language. Sadly, these results have had marginal impact on true interoperability, and many gaps persist. Fortunately, interface engines have been created to narrow the gap. These third-party integration services facilitate data exchange between EHRs and telemedicine systems. Instead of integrating with hundreds of EHRs, telemedicine apps can integrate with an interface engine, which handles the integration to EHRs. While helpful, these services are an added expense and require management.

Regardless of the type of EHR integration needed, any data integration will require significant effort on the part of your health IT team. You need to justify why integration is so important to your organization and whether it's even worth the effort. A several-month effort to simply display a patient name in the telemedicine app probably isn't worth the time or money. It's always worth asking: Why use data integration? Is it necessary? What problem does it solve? Is it worth the effort? Is there an easier way to do it? While EHR integration is nice to have, the benefit might not be worth the effort.

> **While EHR integration is nice to have, the benefit might not be worth the effort.**

Finally, it's worth noting that not all telemedicine systems are designed to collect or use patient data; instead, many focus on delivering real-time audio-visual communication and leave the patient health data recording and storing functions to the EHR. In such cases, sometimes it's easier to manually record the information or use the patient portal to upload and exchange information.

The EHR is at the center of the clinical workflow, and to be successful with telemedicine, you must understand and define what you mean by EHR "integration." Start with relatively easy workflow integrations between your EHR and telehealth solution. If data can be shared between systems, determine whether it's worth the effort; if it is, find the easiest way to do it.

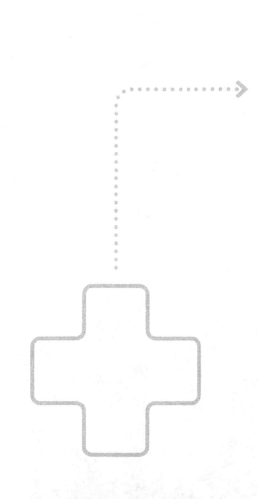

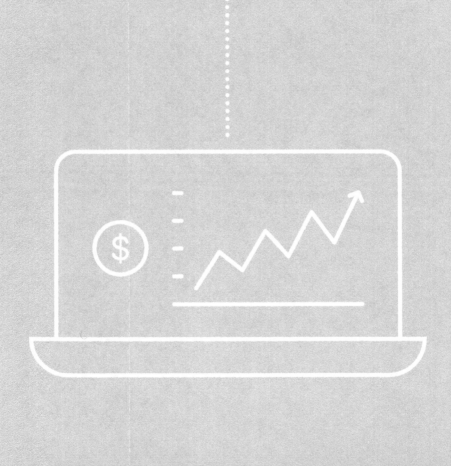

Financial Success

The modern US healthcare industry is a confusing mix of payment models, all with their own strengths, weaknesses, quirks, and rules. As a result, reimbursement remains one of the most popular and complicated topics within telehealth and remains one of biggest barriers to its widespread adoption. We could write an entire book on the various payment models and reimbursement policies for telehealth, but given the constant pace of change, everything would be obsolete by the time this book goes to press. In spite of this, there are still many ways to get paid for providing telehealth services, and for telehealth to be successful, it must be financially feasible for clinicians. This section will help you understand how to navigate the opportunities that exist.

Remuneration for medical services has been ubiquitous throughout history. More often than not, the patient or their family would be expected to pay. Some ancient temples provided healing services in exchange for sacrifices, prayers, and/or donations. Many churches supported infirmaries with nuns tasked with caring for the sick and dying as an act of benevolence. Kings would often hire doctors to care for them and their courts, and later, wealthy landowners would pay doctors to treat their servants and slaves. In some communities, doctors would be hired and paid from some form of tax.

As the world emerged from the Industrial Revolution, urbanized populations and organized labor created new models of healthcare remuneration. In the early American republic, large railroads and logging companies would even provide free healthcare to preserve their investment in their employees and promote efficiency. The earliest forms of health insurance were more like modern disability insurance, which paid specific, predetermined amounts for accidental injuries on railroads or steamboats; they were mostly put in place to cover the loss of wages due to injury or sickness, since the lost wages were usually greater than the cost of medical care itself.

Before the twentieth century, healthcare was still in a rudimentary state, so it was not very expensive. In the early 1900s, several factors led to an increase in the cost of providing medical care. First, the growing professionalization of medicine led to the implementation of strict professional standards and a limited supply of licensed professionals, which drove up costs. Additionally, advances in medical technology and the centralization of medicine around urban hospitals further increased the cost of providing care.

The first precursor to modern health insurance came in 1929, when a group of Dallas teachers contracted with Baylor University Hospital to provide twenty-one days of hospitalization for a fixed payment of fifty cents (approximately $7 today when adjusted for inflation). The arrangement gained traction because it provided the hospital with a constant stream of revenue during the Great Depression and allowed the patient to affordably pay for their care. As this schema became increasingly popular, community hospitals began to band together to reduce competition with one another. Eventually, they came to call themselves Blue Cross. In turn, physicians created their own plans and ultimately affiliated in 1946 as Blue Shield.

Since there was a clear benefit to low-income individuals, states allowed many health insurers to act as nonprofit corporations, which exempted them from taxes. Without this special treatment, it's unlikely the health insurance model would have survived its early years. Eventually, however, commercial insurance companies started to package health insurance along with their other life and property insurance products. Because they weren't bound by state laws and could customize their premiums based upon age and health, they were able to undercut and overtake the market.

World War II profoundly shaped the health insurance industry. As the war tightened the labor market and government restricted wage increases, health insurance became a popular, tax-exempt fringe benefit to attract potential employees. As a result, the number of people enrolled in health insurance plans grew from under 20 million to over 130 million between 1940 and 1960, where three-quarters of Americans had some form of health insurance.[200]

For decades, many advocated for the government to implement nationalized health insurance, but it was consistently rejected due to fears of socialism encroaching into healthcare. As a result, employer-sponsored insurance became firmly established as the dominant way to pay for healthcare in the US. In 1965 Congress passed the Medicare and Medicaid acts as extensions of the Social Security Act, largely to fill the gap of uninsured left out of employer-based health insurance, whether due to age, disability, or inability to work. Though the Medicare and Medicaid acts were signed together, and the organizations were centralized within the Centers of Medicare and Medicaid

Services (CMS), they serve different purposes and have different eligibility requirements to this day.

Medicare is a federal program that covers those who are over sixty-five, have a disability or debilitating chronic disease, or have a number of other conditions. Coverage is the same regardless of state, and the program is funded through payroll taxes and Congress-authorized funds. Medicaid, by comparison, is a joint federal and state program that provides coverage principally for those with limited incomes and resources, individuals with disabilities, terminally ill patients, children, and pregnant women. While there are federal rules, each state runs its own Medicaid program.

As advances in medical research and technology created new ways to diagnose and treat patients, previously untreatable diseases became treatable. As patients lived longer, they cost more to care for, and healthcare became a victim of its own success. Meanwhile, the traditional fee-for-service reimbursement model, where clinicians are reimbursed for each service they provide, increasingly incentivized clinicians to offer more services to patients. As a result, healthcare costs started to rise substantially in the 1970s.

> **As patients lived longer, they cost more to care for, and healthcare became a victim of its own success.**

CMS initially agreed to reimburse physicians at a "usual, customary, and reasonable rate." But as Medicare expenditures rose dramatically, CMS had to make major changes in reimbursement policies. In the early 1980s, CMS capped and fixed hospital reimbursement rates for inpatient hospital services. A tidal wave of changes in the healthcare industry followed.

First came a shift from hospital-based services toward outpatient-based services, which were not restricted by capped reimbursement rates. As a result, the number of outpatient clinics grew from 200 in 1983 to more than 1,500 in 1991. The percentage of surgeries performed in hospitals was roughly halved between 1980 and 1992, from 83.7 percent to 46.1 percent, as the percentage of hospitals with outpatient care departments grew from 50 percent to 87 percent. Hospital revenues derived from outpatient services also doubled, reaching 25 percent of all revenues by 1992.[201]

Additionally, since the new price cap was set exclusively for Medicare payments, hospitals began to shift unreimbursed costs to private health insurance plans. As a result, the average cost of an employee health plan premium more than doubled between 1984 and 1991. When health insurance costs started to affect company profits, many employers sought to reduce costs and did so by reducing plan benefits and requiring employees to pay a larger share of their premiums or copays in turn.

Many employers also turned to lower-priced managed care plans to provide a check against runaway healthcare costs. These plans sought to keep costs low by eliminating unnecessary expenditures through selectively contracting with "in-network" providers, who were willing to offer their services at discounted rates. They also used primary care providers as gatekeepers to care, frequently redirecting patients toward lower-cost services and requiring prior authorization for certain medical interventions or procedures.

By the early 1990s, the majority of those receiving health insurance through their employers did so via managed care plans. In the early days, some managed care practices were excessive and frequently entailed convoluted requirements, denial of medically necessary services, and overly restrictive limits on hospital stays. The resulting public outcry led to the passage of *hundreds* of laws intended to protect patient rights and govern managed care practices throughout the 1990s.

In the meantime, both Medicare and Medicaid expanded their eligibility, allowing more people access to government-funded healthcare. By the turn of the century, Medicare and Medicaid accounted for one-third of all healthcare expenditures in the US. At the same time, roughly 14 percent of Americans still lacked a form of private or government-funded health insurance. In response, the Affordable Care Act (ACA) was passed in 2009, which introduced subsidies for patients and expanded the Medicaid program to cover all adults with income below 138 percent of the federal poverty level. At the time of writing, the uninsured rate now hovers around 8 percent.

The ACA also implemented a variety of healthcare delivery system reforms, including federal recognition of the accountable care organization (ACO). There are many variations of ACOs, but the model generally aligns the payer and clinician under the same organization and ties reimbursements to healthcare outcomes. It also moves reimbursement from a fee-for-service model to a bundled payment model, which groups all services rendered into a particular *episode* of care; for example, a bundled payment for knee replacement surgery would cover preoperative consultations, the surgery itself, postoperative care, and rehabilitation.

The bundled payment model incentivizes clinicians to provide high-quality care while minimizing unnecessary costs. To do this, these organizations typically invest more resources in preventive care, evidence-based disease management, and efficient care coordination. Kaiser Permanente, Intermountain, and Geisinger have been doing this for years and are consistently cited as examples of how to provide high-quality care at below-average cost.[202]

Value-based care is becoming increasingly popular for the cost-savings potential. Meanwhile, a report from 2021 found that 87 percent of company executives believe healthcare costs will become unsustainable within five to ten years.[203] As a result, consolidation of payers and providers into a single organization is the current trend in healthcare, and the past decade has seen a larger number of insurance companies aligning with care organizations. For example, the insurer UnitedHealthcare runs a provider subsidiary called OptumCare, and the pharmacy CVS Health acquired insurer Aetna—a trend we expect to see more of in the future.

In this section, we'll focus less on the constantly changing *policies* and more on broader *motivators* of payers, as well as the levers one can pull to successfully receive reimbursement for telehealth. For better or worse, the government is the biggest driver of policy changes in the healthcare industry, so we'll start with Medicaid and Medicare (chapter 11). From there, we'll discuss government-funded programs outside of the US that have been used to pay for telehealth around the world (chapter 12). Private payers often follow the lead of government payers, so it's also worth exploring private payer models in greater detail (chapter 13). And finally, because financial success goes beyond reimbursement, we'll explore how telehealth can help organizations reduce costs and increase market share (chapter 14).

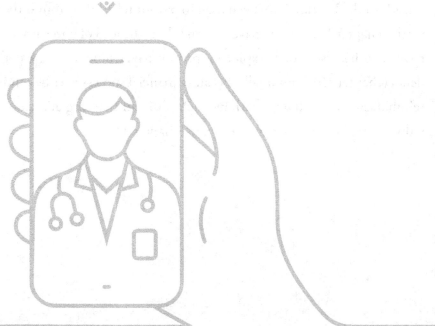

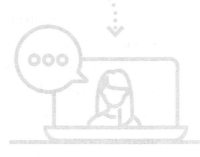

CHAPTER 11

Medicaid and Medicare

Aditi U. Joshi

To be successfully reimbursed for telemedicine from Medicare and Medicaid, it's necessary to understand the key differences between the two. Medicare is designed to cover people who are over sixty-five or are living with disabilities, debilitating chronic diseases, and/or a variety of other conditions. Medicare has doubled the number of patients over sixty-five that have health insurance and has decreased the financial burden for the senior population.[204]

Medicare has an outsized influence on healthcare reimbursement policy. Though it

> **Medicare has an outsized influence on healthcare reimbursement policy.**

covers a smaller percentage of the population than other payers, it is the largest payer for inpatient care, primarily due to the elderly and sick populations it covers. As a result, when Medicare expands policies or sets a payment, other payers tend to follow suit. By setting de facto reimbursement standards for guidelines, payment policy, and regulations, Medicare effectively acts as a unified cost containment force for the American health system at large.

Medicare is divided into different parts. Part A covers hospital care, and Part B covers outpatient services (and whatever's not covered by Part A). Parts C and D are optional and require extra funding. Part C, a.k.a. Medicare Advantage, funds a private insurer to cover enrollees. Part D covers prescriptions and includes MediGap, a bridge insurance program that works with private insurance to handle items that don't fall under general coverage.

Medicaid, on the other hand, is for vulnerable populations, such as those with limited resources, disabilities, the terminally ill, children (CHIP), and pregnant women. Overall, the program has been successful: those with Medicaid in childhood have fewer emergency visits and hospitalizations later in life, better educational attainment, and reduced teen mortality.[205]

Because Medicaid is still under the CMS umbrella, there are federal rules that Medicaid programs must follow, but each state technically runs their own programs under their own names. States must cover certain services through their Medicaid programs, including doctor visits; hospital visits; and mental health, prenatal and maternity care, and preventive care. Aside from those guidelines, eligibility and benefits for other services vary by state as long as they don't conflict with superseding federal laws. Naturally, this makes Medicaid coverage and reimbursement more complicated than Medicare.

For clinicians to become eligible for reimbursement from Medicare, they need to apply for an NPI (National Provider Identifier) through their regional Medicare office. With a few exceptions, to obtain an NPI, one must generally either be a physician, nurse, pharmacist, physical therapist, psychologist, dentist, or chiropractor—or work for a lab, health maintenance organization, hospital, ambulance company, or pharmacy. By comparison, to become a Medicaid provider, you have to apply within every state you want to cover, and sometimes even within a district, which becomes especially complicated for those who are practicing telehealth across state lines.[h]

Once a practitioner is approved, Medicare billing is fairly straightforward, though not always at the level some would like. Medicare sets prices through a set fee schedule for clinicians, as well as a list of costs for other common services, including ambulance, labs, medical equipment, supplies, orthotics, and beyond. After a service or procedure has been rendered, five-digit Current Procedural Terminology (CPT®) codes are used to identify services for billing and reporting purposes. Conversely, Medicaid billing is state-specific but has similar processes and requirements to Medicare.

To bill using a particular code, the medical record documentation must reflect the corresponding level of care. For example, for a clinician delivering critical care services to an ER patient who wants to add a CPT code on the corresponding bill, the documentation has to include evidence to support that claim, including the amount of time spent providing undivided care to that patient. If documentation *doesn't* support the criteria of critical care, that clinician cannot bill for those services provided.

On top of this, providers that bill Medicare need to keep up with annual changes in fee schedules. In turn, they need to be constantly trained and retrained on how to bill correctly. As a result, an entire ecosystem has developed to support billing, coding, reimbursement,

---

h   See chapter 21.

and documentation. Of course, this is all exceedingly complicated, and a lot of work; the administrative overhead is one of the many reasons American healthcare costs are so high.

Telehealth before Covid

While NASA was using telehealth to connect with astronauts in orbit as early as the 1960s, CMS was one of the first government organizations to use telehealth for patients outside of aerospace and the military; it has been reimbursing telehealth services since 2002. Their expansion was slow and deliberate, and their efforts have helped to establish telehealth's foundation, particularly with respect to regulatory laws and the expansion of access.

Medicare has always tended toward caution and cost containment and has approached telehealth reimbursement and policy in a predictably conservative way. Early on, payments were restricted to rural and Health Professional Shortage Areas (HPSAs), where people, hospitals, and clinics were scarce. Reimbursement was further restricted to only certain types of clinicians: physicians, nurse practitioners, physician assistants, midwives, psychologists, social workers, or registered dieticians. Asynchronous telehealth was not covered, so images or chats were not included in coverage.

Additionally, there were restrictions on where a given patient happened to be *sitting* while doing a telehealth visit, which was called an "originating site." Initially, the originating site for patients had to be within some type of healthcare facility, whether a physician's office, a rural health clinic, hospital, skilled nursing facility, or other health center—but *not* from their homes.

Most of these regulations were set up to help expand telehealth access, but their complicated nature ultimately hindered it, especially as the technology advanced. The restrictions created confusion among providers, most of whom would rather bill patients directly than deal with CPT codes, originating sites, documentation, and restrictions. In the end, the headache and uncertainty created by all of the restrictions led many to leave a substantial amount of Medicare money on the table. Between 2008 and 2016, telehealth visits grew from 0.81 to 5.23 per 1,000 patients, which only represents 0.5 percent of all visits reimbursed.[206] The most common beneficiaries were under sixty-five, disabled, dual Medicare/Medicaid eligible, and living in rural areas.[i]

Then, as the federal perception of telehealth started to change, the CONNECT (Creating Opportunities Now for Necessary & Effective Care Technologies) Act was introduced in 2016. This legislation sought to significantly expand Medicare telehealth coverage by removing geographic restrictions and expanding originating sites to include patients' homes. Despite bipartisan and broad external support, it was never passed, even after several attempts at reintroduction.

Crucially, the CONNECT Act still managed to produce a framework for how telehealth reimbursement and care could be expanded, and it continued to inform subsequent legislation. CMS has expanded telehealth in intervals ever since. In 2017, many Medicare patients could choose to include telehealth visits as part of their care, and in 2018, certain patients with chronic conditions could opt for telehealth instead of an in-person follow-up, though they were still required to be seen in person every three months. Overall, changes were slow in coming, and most efforts aimed at expanding telehealth failed to take hold until the pandemic hit.

---

i   A common misconception was that all distant physician encounters "counted" as telehealth, which wasn't true. Radiologists and pathologists, who also provided remote services, were considered "physician services" and not telehealth despite being lumped into the same statistics, so the actual numbers of what we'd truly consider telehealth were likely even lower.

MEDICAID

Despite falling under the CMS umbrella, Medicaid has had a slightly different trajectory in relation to telehealth. Because Medicaid programs are state specific, each state could determine what type of telehealth services were reimbursed, and for what amounts. As early as 2015, forty-six of the fifty states had various telehealth services covered by Medicaid—thirty-six allowed primary care, seventeen allowed text-based communication, and sixteen even allowed for physical and occupational therapy to be delivered over telehealth.

This created a wide array of parity laws, which predate Covid, and are a common topic of discussion in the telehealth industry. *Parity* essentially refers to what is or isn't considered *equal or comparable* care; in terms of telehealth, the primary distinction is between remote and in-person visits. If a law determines telehealth to be equal or comparable to in-person care, they've effectively stated that telehealth *is* a viable and equal type of healthcare service modality, and payment parity should ostensibly follow close behind.

Telehealth parity is further divided into *payment parity* and *service parity*, and the latter does not guarantee the same rate of payment. Each state has different parity laws, which is where things continue to get even more complicated. Any given state may offer payment parity, service parity, or both, and how much each state pays influences how laws are written, as well as how payment works via Medicaid *and* private insurance.

By 2020, many Medicaid programs were expanding telehealth coverage to certain patients in rural and underserved areas. The aim was to improve access, reduce costs, and most importantly, to distribute care more equitably to vulnerable populations, many of whom struggle to find clinicians who accept Medicaid. Because Medicaid telehealth expansion varied by state, it ultimately became an easy way to test and compare results between states. For example, one study found that states that had Medicaid expansion had 54 percent more telemental health claims than those that did not.[207] In those where private insurers paid for telehealth, adoption rates were much higher than in states that didn't.[208]

Overall, Medicaid beneficiaries had more flexibility in terms of using telehealth as compared to Medicare, but state restrictions continued to impact what programs they could use and their overall outcomes, paving the way for many of the changes that came about during and after the pandemic.

CMS Telehealth Expansion during Covid

The trajectory of telehealth within CMS changed overnight with Covid, principally through the passing of the $2.2 trillion CARES (Coronavirus Aid, Relief, and Economic Security) Act in March 2020. While most of the package was related to preventing the economic fallout of Covid, the act also included provisions aimed at improving Covid-related healthcare, including vaccine development, testing, treatment, resource allocation, and an expansion of telehealth services in Medicare.

It brought about the largest-ever sea change in telehealth policy, especially in regard to reimbursement. Clinicians could suddenly bill Medicare for treatment and waive cost-sharing for telehealth visits, which meant that patients no longer had to pay copays or deductibles. Even though telehealth wasn't always paid at the same rates, it *was* paid, which was an enormous change. New patients were now able to receive telehealth care without having a previously established relationship. The "originating site" restrictions were also removed, and clinicians, from their own homes, were free to see patients. Coverage expanded from rural areas to everywhere.

The act's waivers also expanded who was permitted to deliver telehealth, including social workers, psychologists, and physical and occupational therapists, among others. For emergency department patients, medical screening exams could even be conducted via tele-health. Reimbursement for remote patient monitoring, mental health, and chronic care expanded, as did telephone visits, which increased access for seniors without internet connections.

> **There were 52.7 million total Medicare telehealth visits in 2020, compared to 840,000 in 2019—a staggering sixty-three-fold increase.**

As a result of these changes, the CARES Act dramatically increased the use of telehealth. In April 2020, nearly half (43.5 percent or 1.28 million per week) of Medicare primary care visits were conducted via telemedicine, compared to only 0.1 percent two months prior. By the summer and fall of 2020, more than 25 percent of Medicare beneficiaries had had a telehealth visit. There were 52.7 million total telehealth visits in 2020, compared to 840,000 in 2019—a staggering sixty-three-fold increase.[209] Notably, telehealth use was highest among Medicare beneficiaries with long-term dis-abilities, Black and Hispanic populations, and those with multiple conditions, all of which are populations that telehealth would benefit the most.[210]

Medicaid expanded just as quickly as Medicare during the pandemic, but the state-specific nature of Medicaid made some of the resulting changes predictably more complicated. The federal emergency waivers declared that there was parity between telehealth and in-person care nationwide; however, each state could decide which type of parity they were delivering, whether service or payment. Physicians still had to hold a license in the states in which their patients were located, and in the beginning of the pandemic, restrictions were relaxed so clinicians could continue seeing patients across state lines, despite varying rules from state to state.[j]

All of this contributed to hectic adoption and rollout. Primary care practices identified reimbursement confusion as a top barrier to telehealth use,[211] and many clinics struggled with telehealth implementation.[212] To alleviate some of this confusion, the CMS created a Telehealth Toolkit, which provided information on regulations, barriers, reimbursement, and what state was generally doing what, but its utility was limited, and few gained value from it.[213]

As the pandemic waned, the number of telehealth visits among Medicare beneficiaries correspondingly fell. As a result, some of the telehealth initial expansions have expired, or are set to expire, while others have been continuously extended. In turn, Medicaid has expanded in some ways and backed off in others. Covid-era waivers will change significantly in the coming years, but the forward movement of telehealth within Medicare during the pandemic and beyond cannot be ignored.

The Future of Telehealth and CMS

Given the enormity of the aging population in the US, CMS financial success will depend on increased telehealth use. The future of telehealth with CMS is complicated to predict, but the government has shown that they are willing to continuously extend many of their

---

j   See chapter 21 for more detailed analysis of how changing state laws during the pandemic affected reimbursement.

recent changes to keep telehealth in effect. The question is: For how long? In December of 2022, the government passed the Omnibus Bill, which extends telehealth flexibilities until the end of 2024. Then, in January 2023, President Biden announced that the public health emergency waivers would end on May 11 of the same year. While these appear to be at odds with one another, the Omnibus Bill has introduced some of the waivers into a federal spending bill, effectively decoupling them from the emergency waivers. In other words, even when the emergency waivers go away, many of their telehealth reimbursements and flexibilities will remain.

For example, Medicare beneficiaries in any geographic area can still receive care and can do so from their homes, and many of the reimbursed and covered services will be covered by the omnibus bill and will not expire. On the other hand, some copays may likely come back without the waivers. There are also administrative changes. For example, Medicare now requires doctors to fill out a form for their homes and offices if both are being used for telehealth.

Medicaid, as always, is more complicated to predict because each state can determine what they want to do going forward. Many states have already made some Medicaid telehealth flexibilities permanent or are planning to.[214] For example, Michigan is planning to eliminate coverage of audio-only services while keeping the codes intact, so those needing behavioral health counseling with limited broadband can still access care. New York is planning on making audio-only visit coverage permanent. Ohio has expanded telehealth coverage for pregnancy, diabetes, and behavioral health, while South Carolina is planning on decreasing some of their behavioral health service coverage.

It's all quite difficult to keep up with, even for those who work in this field. A national group that I am part of was tasked with creating CPT codes and codifying billing for digital medicine and telehealth. At one of the meetings, a specialist in CMS codes about reimbursement updated us on changes in response to emergency waiver changes. When the group had several questions about what was going to happen next, even the presenter herself wasn't sure of how to answer many of them.

Medicare and Medicaid are major healthcare payers in the US, and as a result, both are strong influencers of telehealth reimbursement. While permanent changes to telehealth are largely incumbent on Congress, there are a few things we can do to be successful. First, it's important to understand CMS reimbursement policies and follow them. If you accept CMS, stay up to date on the changing rules and requirements and ensure your reimbursements are compliant. Second, continue to use telehealth services whenever they're available, and bill for what you can. When services fall out of use, they're more likely to be cut. CMS aggregates telehealth-related utilization and results, including cost effectiveness and impact, and uses them to convince legislators and lawmakers to extend telehealth beyond the pandemic.[215] Finally, lobby and advocate for telehealth reimbursement to continue where you can, and at all levels. As the federal government sets the tone for states and the rest of the healthcare industry, doing this will help further solidify telehealth in the broader firmament of American healthcare.

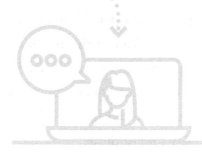

CHAPTER 12

Government-Led Healthcare

F unding healthcare is expensive, especially when you consider doing so for a nation's entire population. Healthcare is also an economic good, and governments worldwide recognize the economic value of health for their citizens, from bolstering life expectancy, to prolonging healthy working years, to increasing population growth, and more. In turn, governments have a hand in balancing the public's infinite need for healthcare with the healthcare industry's finite resources and capacity to provide it.[216]

Though all governments handle this task differently, healthcare models generally fall into four categories based on who's paying for it and who's supplying it. First, there's a single-payer system, where a national health service both supplies and funds the services, such as the NHS in the UK or the Veterans Health Administration in the US. Next, there's single-payer national health insurance, where the government pays, but healthcare providers are private, as in Canada, or American Medicare. Third, there's the Bismarck or "social health insurance" model, where private insurers fund healthcare while the government regulates prices, as in Germany and France. Finally, there's the out-of-pocket model, which is how many developing countries pay for healthcare.

In reality, these models are not ubiquitous in each country, and most nations see a combination of these four models. In India, patients typically pay out of pocket but occasionally have insurance. The NHS in the UK is free at the point of care, yet many are willing to pay more for private insurance to get quicker care at a private practice.

In this chapter, we'll look at various government reimbursement models and examine how they've respectively influenced the adoption of telehealth. We'll also examine a few international case studies to understand how and why different incentives around the world have variously contributed and inhibited the growth of telemedicine, as each offers clues to how telehealth will develop in the future.

US Models

The American healthcare system is one of the most complicated in the world; it encompasses a wide variety of payment models and isn't broadly transparent in terms of data, outcomes, or reimbursements. American healthcare's reputation as a capitalistic, private, insurance-led health system tends

> **The American healthcare system is one of the most complicated in the world.**

to overshadow the fact that large, centralized government programs within its borders also exist. While each of these programs is unique, they all use telehealth to help with cost containment, and in equally unique ways.

VETERANS ADMINISTRATION

The Veterans Administration (VA) was formed after World War I prompted Congress to establish a system of programs for disability compensation. It's gone through a few iterations over the decades, but today, the VA functions as a unique, specialized, single-payer system whose annual budget must be approved by Congress. Its facilities are entirely owned and operated by the federal government, which makes their model more similar to the UK's NHS than anything else stateside.

Telehealth is ideal for the VA because their hospitals are primarily located near major cities, and recent closures of hospitals have added to a growing gap in access. Additionally, veterans tend to require specialized services, particularly for disabilities and post-traumatic stress disorder (PTSD). By 2013, the VA had already seen over six hundred thousand patients via telehealth, and by 2016, over nine hundred VA sites were implementing telehealth over fifty specialties. During the pandemic, their Video Connect program expanded even further, decreasing hospitalizations and ER visits. VA telehealth visits per month increased between February and May of 2020 from 10,000 to 120,000—an astonishing 1,000 percent increase.[217]

> **VA telehealth visits per month increased between February and May of 2020 from 10,000 to 120,000—an astonishing 1,000 percent increase.**

Historically travel reimbursements have been one of the VA's largest expenses. One evaluation found that telehealth led to an 82.5 percent reduction in missed appointments with an estimated cost savings in travel reimbursements of $3,308.30.[218] Telemedicine volume grew so significantly over one study period that by its final year, the travel pay savings had increased to $63,804, or about 3.5 percent of the total travel pay disbursement for that year.[219]

Because the VA has centralized medical records, they were one of the early leaders in telehealth research, particularly in terms of examining cost savings and outcomes. VA telemedicine patients have lower utilization costs and found their care to be on par with in-person care.[220] On top of saving on travel reimbursements, a single VA pain clinic also reduced their missed appointments by 80 percent by using telehealth.[218] Various VA studies have also noted that telemedicine leads to greater cost savings and improvement in PTSD care.[221] As the VA endures one budget cut after another, telemedicine stands to become more and more important for their cause.

TRICARE

TRICARE is a government-funded managed health insurance program for the military, retirees, and their family members. TRICARE offers a number of diverse insurance plans, and most resemble commercial insurance plans. Those eligible can use Department of Defense–operated military hospitals and clinics as well as in-network and Tricare-authorized civilian clinicians. Because low reimbursement rates limit where enrollees can access clinicians and get care in civilian areas, telemedicine has become an increasingly important solution for this population. TRICARE covers video and audio telemedicine as a stand-in for in-office visits, preventive health, mental health, and end-stage renal disease. TRICARE is also among the only insurance services to have made audio-only telemedicine a permanent benefit, and even has its own telehealth platform, MHS Video Connect. Since many TRICARE recipients have dual insurance with commercial payers, Medicare, and others, TRICARE is increasingly partnering with direct-to-consumer (DTC) telemedicine companies like Doctor on Demand.

There have been some hiccups in the process. In 2019, TRICARE telehealth claims were $4 million, and by September 2020, they'd ballooned to $150 million. Due to the general chaos of the pandemic, TRICARE found they'd overpaid on telehealth claims, money that could have been used elsewhere; their example highlights how important it is to have the right team around to keep up with expenditures and policy changes.[222]

INDIAN HEALTH SERVICES

Indian Health Services (IHS), a federal agency of the Department of Health and Human Services, formed to serve the health needs of Native Americans and Alaska Natives within the US. The IHS is not health insurance; it's a health *budget* intended to cover health services and programs via clinics, hospitals, health centers, and community centers. Similar to the VA, the IHS is required to submit annual budgets for review by the House and Senate. The IHS budget is not sufficient to comprehensively cover all health needs, so beneficiaries often supplement with other forms of insurance such as Medicaid.

The history of racism, inequality in education, and general poverty have all contributed to high health disparities among the Native American population in comparison to the wider American population, including a lower life expectancy, more chronic disease and malignant cancers, and higher rates of violence, all of which increase healthcare costs. Additionally, most Native Americans live in rural areas, so most are unlikely to be close to an IHS hospital.

For all of these reasons, IHS has been an earlier pioneer of telehealth adoption. Alaskan natives have been using telehealth, particularly store-and-forward, since as early as 2001. One notable project for ear, nose, and throat doctors offered patients same-day consults, and most took less than six minutes. All told, the effort saved Alaska Medicaid $3.1 million.[223] Each $1 spent on this telehealth program saved $11.50 in travel costs. The program remains one of the few that makes clear the cost effectiveness of store-and-forward telehealth for specialty care in large, rural areas.

These cost savings encouraged IHS to invest even more in telehealth expansion, principally by offering specialty services in areas that were only previously equipped to offer primary care, including diabetes, substance use disorder, and sexually transmitted diseases. Previously, many IHS patients faced formidable travel barriers to receive specialty care, and by expanding telehealth, the program saved approximately one billion dollars over three years.[k] As the IHS continues to expand its telehealth services, poor internet connectivity and device access in many of these tribal areas remain barriers. At the time of writing, the High Speed Internet for All program has encouragingly set aside $7 billion of its $65 billion budget to expand internet services in tribal communities.[224]

International Case Studies

Over time, every nation of the world has developed its own unique way of providing and funding healthcare, and most continue to

---

k   Interview with Justin Fultcher, CEO of telemedicine company RingMD, which IHS used.

develop equally unique approaches to telehealth. In this section, we'll examine a few of the more striking examples from around the world, as their respective successes and failures are equally instructive.

BANGLADESH

In resource-limited countries, quality healthcare tends to be hard to access. Bangladesh has a highly decentralized healthcare model and a mixed system of public and private financing, which entails significant out-of-pocket expenses for patients, as well as a high reliance on external aid, NGOs, for-profit companies, and the national government. Their population of 170 million is served through government-run hospitals and privately run clinics, where the length of an average patient-doctor visit is forty-eight seconds, only four labs nationwide meet international standards, and more than 20 percent of the drugs are counterfeit.

In the midst of all of this, Sylvana Q. Sinha believed that better, more accessible healthcare in Bangladesh was possible and that telehealth was the key. Sinha compensated for her limited budget by focusing on what she herself could fix and concentrating on best practices and successful use cases from around the world. Today, her company, Praava Health, employs a hybrid model that emphasizes continuity of care and combines telehealth access with a full suite of in-clinic offerings, including in-house primary and secondary care, outpatient procedures, lab and imaging diagnostics, and pharmacy. Using Praava, patients who required labs or radiology tests for diagnosis could receive those orders via telehealth rather than needing to find a separate clinic or lab themselves.

Her model succeeded. Praava's first clinic reached an operating breakeven within ten months, and their model currently boasts 60+ percent gross margins. To date, they've helped nearly half a million people, all while increasing patient retention and satisfaction *and* maintaining high quality and efficiency. Achieving similar results, even in challenging environments, doesn't have to be expensive, especially if we learn from others' mistakes. Now similar hybrid models are seeing similar success all over the world.[225, 226]

THE UNITED KINGDOM

The UK's National Health Services (NHS) is the most well-known example of a single payer and provider in the world. Their system has been an example to the world in a variety of ways, and the first lesson is this: free, government-staffed healthcare for all is expensive to administer. The NHS workforce is also plagued by burnout, clinician shortages, overburdened hospitals, and overwhelming patient loads—all of which were exacerbated by the pandemic. Long waits for care are also common, whether for routine checkups, nonemergent procedures, or specialist consultations. In response, private insurance companies have flourished in the UK because they offer drastically reduced wait times, private hospital rooms—perks that widen health disparities.

This situation has created unique opportunities for telehealth, especially in terms of improving access and reducing costs. Even before the pandemic, the NHS sought to save £1.2 billion over a period of five years through increased use of telehealth and increasingly made a concerted effort to be "digital first." In the process, they sought for all primary care practices to have an online presence, phase out fax machines, enable online access to patient medical records, and offer telehealth visits when appropriate. This gained considerable momentum during and after the pandemic. In 2020, outpatient telephone and video consults went from 4 percent to 35 percent of their overall volume in April alone.

Perhaps the most interesting aspect of healthcare in the UK involves the deep complexities and unintended consequences of intermingling for-profit and not-for-profit entities; one well-known case is particularly illustrative. A general practitioner (GP) practice partnered with a for-profit company called Babylon Health to provide virtual care in a district of London. The online practice was called GP at Hand. Normally, patients within the NHS are assigned a GP within their local region, and each practice is given a corresponding budget allocation for their patient population. GP at Hand essentially functioned like a normal GP practice, but—and this is a large but—without the normal geographical restrictions of one, as it was entirely virtual.

As patients generally favored the convenience of finding a GP via telehealth, an exodus of approximately four thousand patients a month began leaving their existing practices and streamed into a new, virtual practice. Initially, this seemed like a win for telehealth, and then a host of unintended consequences followed. First, patients and NHS funding were diverted away from competing practices, causing concern that GP at Hand was cherry-picking younger, healthier patients and leaving the NHS with sicker, more costly ones.[227] At the time, its patient population definitely skewed young—85 percent were between twenty and thirty-nine years old, despite that same demographic comprising only 28 percent of the overall population.[228] As GP at Hand swelled to ten times its original size, the disruptions that followed were met by on-the-street protests from patients, many of whom hadn't realized they'd deregistered from their local practice in the process of signing on.[229] Many suddenly found it hard to see a doctor and tried going back to their old in-person clinics, with enormous confusion on all sides as a result.

In short, the machinations of a private company posed serious challenges to how the entire government system functioned, illustrating the extent to which it's necessary to ensure that your telehealth goals are aligned with whom you're doing business with—especially when one party's ultimate aim is for profit and the other's isn't. The NHS continues to innovate and pilot digital-first programs, and in the end, the most successful of them pursued clear, aligned financial goals and were agile enough to pivot when necessary.

> **The machinations of a private company posed serious challenges to how the entire government system functioned.**

SINGAPORE

Based on life expectancy, maternal mortality, efficiency, and outcomes, Singapore's healthcare system is among the best in the world. Moreover, its system comprises 3 percent of their GDP, much less than the US's 20 percent. One-quarter of Singapore's public healthcare system is funded by taxes, with the rest covered by insurance, cost sharing, and a compulsory savings program that resembles American health savings accounts. When patients walk into a Singaporean clinic, they still pay something out of pocket, a system designed to discourage medically unnecessary services. Most, but not all, fees are published and transparent. Patients can go to public or private hospitals, though it's usually cheaper to go to public hospitals. Like most places, Singapore's healthcare costs are rising and will likely continue to do so due to its aging population.

Singapore has attempted to cut costs via broad governmental interventions, regulating its ranks of physicians and negotiating to spend less on drugs. Initially, the government let hospitals freely compete, but this led the hospitals to focus on offering more expensive services, which predictably increased costs and widened access disparities. Once the government discovered that they couldn't just let the market have its way, it stepped in to establish guides and approval processes. The situation is similar to what's transpired in the US: when you let market forces run rampant within healthcare, not only will the market fail, but your population's overall health will broadly worsen.

One of Singapore's most significant telehealth interventions relates to primary care providers. Singapore's primary care network is made up of private practitioners who may house their own medication dispensaries, making profits from care and prescriptions, potentially creating incentives to overprescribe. The government turned to MyDoc, a telemedicine company working regionally, to curtail overprescribing by using a central pharmacy to manage prescriptions as doctors only worked on patient visits. This dropped the antibiotic prescription rates by a whopping 50 percent, significantly lowering costs and improving care overall.

This success persuaded the government to consider a national virtual-first program. In it, a wide spectrum of patients—from those with colds all the way up to those who need surgery—are directed to access telehealth as their first point of contact with the healthcare system. From there, they're directed either toward another telehealth appointment, a clinic, or a hospital. The goal is to streamline care for all and decrease perverse incentives.

Singapore has a few inherent advantages that make it uniquely receptive to telehealth. Its population is generally accepting of innovations in digital health and willing to share data. During the pandemic, for example, Singapore was quick to spring to action on issuing vaccine passports and testing to avoid overwhelming their hospitals. Because much of this was covered by subsidies, it quickly found widespread use.[230]

The most interesting thing about Singapore's case is the unique relationship between the private and public sectors, which has generally created a marketplace that patients tend to like and trust. Much of the country's success with telehealth came from partnerships between startups and the government, whose management of the broader system did *not* lead to market forces taking over and creating skewed incentives—mostly because the government stepped in *before* that happened. Using telehealth first has cut costs, decreased waste and fraud, improved equity and care, and made the Singaporean system agile. This case shows that sensibly merging private and public, keeping incentives focused on health outcomes and equity, and increasing the use of telehealth can all lead to financial success.

GERMANY

Germany's Social Health Insurance (SHI) system is a multipayer system with a high reliance on self-governing structures for regulation. Telehealth has existed in Germany for decades, but it's grown slowly due to regulatory hurdles, most of which are geared toward hitting the nation's clear health policy goals. The first goal is prevention via programs that aim to improve health literacy and promote healthy behaviors. The second is strengthening long-term care by making health at once more individual and adaptable to age-related needs.

To that end, Germany's first eHealth laws went into effect in 2015. At first, telehealth was used only for follow-up appointments. Later, as doctors increasingly recognized barriers to travel, it expanded to general consults, but until the pandemic, doctors were limited to how much time they could spend on telemedicine visits. Online consultations have been allowed in certain instances since 2018, and in 2019, certain visits became billable to SHI. Prepandemic progress was still slow due to the extent of regulations, reimbursement issues, and strict data protections. Then, as in so many other places, the pandemic resulted in relaxed regulations. Most of all, payment parity between telehealth versus in-person visits led to a staggering increase of physicians offering telehealth, from 0.8 percent to 52 percent.[231]

Germany eventually created a centralized digital health application, the DiGA (Digitale Gesundheitsanwendungen), composed of a group of vetted, low-risk medical devices and applications available by prescription. To be vetted and added to the national constellation of health tech, you must first demonstrate improved clinical outcomes, and then, if your device or app doesn't succeed, it's removed from the database. The goal is to have things that work and improve the lives of the population; then, and only then, will they be paid for by the government.

Germany generally focuses heavily on evidence-based outcomes. The high bar to entry has led to high trust among the public and medical professionals. On one hand, Germany is more strict than many other places, to the extent that some have questioned whether they restrict innovation. On the other, they're clear on their goals and consistently ensure that what they're paying for makes sense. To this day, privacy laws are their biggest hurdle for telehealth expansion.

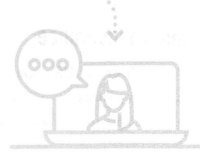

CHAPTER 13

Private Payers

Brandon M. Welch

I n the US, large, for-profit health insurance companies operate with the goal of making money. These companies need to be able to pay claims, cover expenses, and still make a reasonable profit for their shareholders. One way to achieve this is to simply increase premiums, which they've certainly been doing; from 2000 to 2020, insurance premiums have risen from just under $6,000 to over $20,000 a year.[232, 233] On the other hand, they can't simply raise prices beyond what customers can afford. With this in mind, insurers employ a host of other strategies to decrease expenses, including negotiating lower prices for healthcare services and products, preventing unnecessary care and waste, and keeping patients healthy so they don't need to receive healthcare in the first place. If done right, insurers can also use telehealth to avoid unnecessary expenses.

Health Insurance

Over half of the US population is covered under private health insurance, so it stands to reason that telehealth adoption is dependent on private health insurance reimbursement. For this reason, advocates have pushed for insurance companies to reimburse for telehealth. They argued that telemedicine would help insurers avoid high-cost hospital visits, lower morbidity-related costs through increased access to preventative care, and cut down on unnecessary travel costs and hospital transfers that insurers are obligated to pay, among many other things.

> **Over half of the US population is covered under private health insurance.**

Initially, however, insurance companies were resistant. Their primary concern was that patients would utilize telemedicine for common conditions that they would not have otherwise sought treatment for in person, which could lead to higher costs overall. Their concerns weren't unfounded; the 2015 Congressional Budget Office predicted that telemedicine would increase overall spending,[234] and early estimates projected that 90 percent of telemedicine visits would be for care that patients would not have otherwise received without telemedicine.[235]

Additionally, many clinical services, such as follow-up phone visits, were already being provided without being billed for, and insurers would end up spending more by allowing providers to bill for these services. In the end, insurers didn't want providers using telehealth to create new streams of revenue without making patients healthier or reducing their costs. It's very important to remember that insurers are more receptive to paying for clinical services that are *substitutive*—things that will save them money by replacing higher-cost in-person care with lower-cost video visits.

At a broader level, many insurers, concerned about the increased potential for fraud using telehealth,[l] had the impression that the quality of telemedicine was lower than in-person care and feared that it would ultimately lead to greater hospital utilization. For quite some time, they demanded more data to demonstrate cost-effectiveness and quality of care, despite a dearth of comparative research outlining the cost and quality differences between in-person and remote care.

In response, telehealth advocates turned to parity laws to *force* insurers to reimburse for telemedicine.[m] Before the pandemic, thirty-six states required health insurance to cover telemedicine visits but didn't necessarily require that they reimburse *at the same rate*—only fifteen states require insurers to reimburse providers for a telemedicine visit at the same rate. Each state's parity laws came with their own inclusions, exclusions, and requirements–all of which made it frustrating for telehealth providers to navigate the various reimbursement policies across states and insurance companies.

But the fact that a state doesn't have a parity law doesn't necessarily mean parity doesn't already exist. Likewise, insurance companies could choose to reimburse for telehealth without being forced. South Carolina, for example, didn't need parity laws because all health plans in the state had agreed to reimburse for telemedicine. In fact, some insurers were more open to telehealth than in-person care and even updated their billing codes to reimburse for it on their own.

---

l   See chapter 16.

m   Parity laws also discussed in chapter 11.

ADOPTION OF DTC TELEHEALTH SERVICES

Initially, clinicians and patients were hesitant to adopt telehealth, so insurers had little motivation to push for it. As a result, some insurers turned to DTC telemedicine companies, such as Teladoc, Doctor on Demand, and Amwell to provide their members with direct physician access via telehealth. These DTC services are geared mostly toward immediate access to a physician for common, acute, and episodic care issues like colds, rashes, and urinary tract infections. Insurers saw this as a cost-saving opportunity; they understandably wanted to steer patients away from high-cost ER or urgent care visits for simple acute problems.

Unfortunately, despite DTC companies' apparent success as measured by their tens of millions of members, the actual number of DTC *visits* was "pathetically low," according to one health insurance executive.[n] DTC companies cited lack of awareness for low adoption and tried to address the problem through direct mailers, newsletters, marketing campaigns, and listings on the health insurance physician directories, but their efforts had a marginal impact on adoption. Even with services available for a low cost or free, patients simply didn't use it.

Despite providers being easier to access through these services, patients were found to be less comfortable and less willing to use DTC services than meeting with their own provider via telemedicine.[93] Furthermore, in 2015, the American College of Physicians released a position statement recommending that telemedicine should exist "within the context of an established patient-provider relationship in a medical home if it meets the same standards of practice as

---

n   DTC services measure their members as how many covered lives have access to their services as a benefit through their health plan; it is not actual utilization of DTC services.

in-person care." While DTC companies were not trying to displace established patient-provider relationships, this dampened the enthusiasm for DTC telehealth. All the while, insurers continued to retain DTC companies as an urgent care alternative.

IMPACT OF COVID

When Covid hit, health insurers began to see telemedicine as a way to reduce the pandemic's impact along with most everyone else. When Medicare relaxed its own restrictions on reimbursement for telemedicine services, it "strongly encouraged" health insurers to do the same.[236] At the same time, many insurers were concerned that people might avoid seeking treatment due to copay and high deductibles, thereby potentially increasing the spread of Covid. In response, the government passed laws and executive orders *requiring* health plans to waive cost-sharing for Covid-related clinical services.

During the pandemic, insurers were generally cooperative in terms of increasing coverage requirements and relaxing restrictions on telemedicine. In fact, many health insurers started paying for telemedicine services they never expected to, including physical therapy, occupational therapy, and rounding at hospitals. As telemedicine rapidly expanded during the pandemic, reimbursement claims shot up, as did DTC utilization. Then, despite *expanding* coverage to telemedicine, health insurer costs were actually *lower* during the pandemic, mostly because most people generally avoided seeking healthcare unless absolutely necessary.

> **When Covid hit, health insurers began to see telemedicine as a way to reduce the pandemic's impact along with most everyone else.**

As the pandemic waned, health insurers have started pulling back on telemedicine coverage, and with the exceptions of mental and behavioral health, the complaints from consumers have been relatively few. At a broad level, ongoing utilization and demand have been what's kept most postpandemic telehealth reimbursement policies in place. In the meantime, health insurers contend that telemedicine should be reimbursed at a lower rate because of its lower overhead costs compared with in-person services. For now, many health insurers are required to pay the same as in person due to temporary government mandates, but if and when these end, the reimbursed amount may decrease.

NOTABLE VARIATIONS OF HEALTH INSURANCE

Health insurance isn't a monolith. Over 60 percent of people with insurance are covered by employer self-funded plans; in other words, employers opt to pay for claims directly as they arise instead of paying a monthly premium. Self-funded employer plans have greater control over how benefits are spent, including on telehealth. Even before Covid, large employers such as Walmart offered telemedicine as part of their health benefits package.[237] Today, over 95 percent of companies that self-fund cover telemedicine as a health benefit.[238]

Accountable care organizations (ACOs) were also early adopters of telemedicine and have been a leading source for telemedicine cost-effectiveness research ever since. For instance, Kaiser Permanente showed as early as 1996 that home healthcare using telemedicine was more cost-effective than in-person care.[239, 240] Similarly, Geisinger Health conducted a study between 2008 and 2012 that showed that telemonitoring cut readmission rate by 44 percent for heart failure patients—a timely revelation because Medicare stopped reimbursing for care for patients who were readmitted within thirty days in 2012.

ACOs are also incentivized to be innovative with telehealth; for instance, Intermountain Healthcare was quite successful freeing up emergency rooms and hospital beds during Covid using telehealth. They had patients who tested positive for Covid *without* life-threatening symptoms sent home with a Bluetooth pulse oximeter that transmitted their blood oxygen levels to a centrally located nurse care team. If the level was low, a nurse would contact the patient via telehealth to conduct a clinical evaluation. If the patient's condition was found to be severe or deteriorating, they would be sent to the ER. In just over a year, Intermountain handled over ten thousand patients and avoided nearly two thousand unnecessary hospital admissions, all of which freed up beds for critically ill patients at a significant cost savings. Payers don't traditionally reimburse for this kind of remote home monitoring, but because the payer and provider are aligned at Intermountain, they're able to do it.

Self-Pay

Of course, health insurers are far from the only entities struggling to shoulder the rising cost of healthcare. For many reasons, more and more patients are paying out of pocket for their care. As the cost of health insurance continues to rise, more people are moving from traditional insurance plans to high-deductible plans with lower premiums, which cover emergencies and surgeries, while making routine care an out-of-pocket expense.

As a result, many patients are using health savings accounts (HSAs), which allow tax-free contributions that can be used later for deductibles, cost-sharing, and other out-of-pocket medical expenses. These plans are especially popular and advantageous for younger, healthier people who have low healthcare expenses overall. At the time of writing, more than half of Americans under sixty-five are on high-deductible health plans, a rate double that of 2010.[241, 242]

Since self-pay is not reliant on insurance or CMS reimbursement, they are not bound by telehealth restrictions, meaning patients and clinicians tend to pursue the course of action that makes the most sense. As a result, there is a growing number of successful self-pay telehealth services that appeal to patients' demand for convenience, speed, and cost savings, and we expect to see more of these in the future.

CONCIERGE CARE

Concierge medicine, membership care, and direct primary care—where patients typically pay a flat, monthly membership fee for preferential care above and beyond traditional, fee-for-service primary care—is growing. Services often entail more personalized care, including in-depth physical exams, additional screenings, preventative services, lab work, same-day appointments, 24/7 access, and home visits. For major health problems, concierge doctors even coordinate specialist care and hospital visits as necessary. There's a lot of growth and interest in subscription-based healthcare to the extent that Amazon acquired One Medical, a concierge primary care company with seven hundred thousand members, for nearly $4 billion, as part of a broader mission to "reinvent" healthcare.[243]

For their part, concierge providers enjoy the stable income and less in the way of bureaucracy, documentation, overhead, and reimbursement headaches. Also, due to their smaller patient population, they have more time to spend with patients and a better work-life balance. Freed from payer restrictions, concierge providers largely have the freedom to provide care however they see fit. As a result, many have been providing video visits, phone calls, and text messaging to patients for several years. Many concierge providers, such as World

Clinic, have gone entirely virtual, using remote-monitoring technology to take vitals from the patient's home, coordinating blood draws at local medical laboratories, and working with local pharmacies to deliver shots or medications.

The concierge care model is also rapidly growing within the field of mental health. Several companies, including TalkSpace and Betterhelp, offer concierge counseling and mental health services entirely online via telemedicine. For a set price, these concierge mental health services allow patients to meet with a therapist by video, receive prescriptions, and engage in on-demand text-based support to answer questions, change or adjust medication, and track progress.

DIRECT-TO-CONSUMER TELEHEALTH

We've already discussed DTC telehealth in the context of health insurance as a covered benefit, but these services are also available to those willing to pay out of pocket for on-demand services for a wide array of care, including urgent care, primary care, mental health, dermatology, and men's and women's health. There are many variations of the episodic DTC model, each with different models, prices, and offerings. For instance, KHealth offers text-only access to a clinician for questions and prescriptions for $29 per month. Lemonaid similarly partners with mail-order pharmacies and accepts out-of-pocket payment for medications that are shipped directly to the patient's door.

The DTC model also allows clinicians to offer targeted niche care. For example, Joseph Krainin, MD, left his job as a neurologist at a large health system to start SingularSleep, an online sleep clinic that helps people with sleep apnea get CPAP machine prescriptions. His customers were so fed up with the complexity and bureaucracy of in-person sleep evaluations that most were more than happy to pay

$189 to receive a home sleep study test and eventual CPAP prescription, which Krainin also sold and shipped directly to them.°

GetRoman similarly caters to men seeking prescriptions for hair loss and sexual health and bakes the cost of the medical consultation into the cost of the medication they prescribe, which is shipped directly to patients' homes. Cleared to Drive provides New York state driver's license vision tests online for $49, and several online clinics allow patients to meet with certified physicians to obtain medicinal marijuana cards in the states where it's legal. On many additional fronts, telehealth continues to make healthcare easier, cheaper, and more convenient for patients to pay out of pocket for services than going through insurance. As more use this model, it will only continue to grow.

Private payers—whether private insurance, employer-funded, or patients—pay for the bulk of healthcare expenditures in the US. Each payer presents telehealth services with unique opportunities for cost savings. With this in mind, ensure that the telehealth services you're billing for are substitutive and not additive. Use them appropriately, and even more, show that they are saving payers money. Take advantage of using telehealth as part of bundled payments and consider your patients' willingness to self-pay for your telehealth services.

---

o   https://doxy.me/en/resources/podcasts/
     ep-4-bringing-home-better-sleep-with-telemedicine-featuring-dr-joseph-krainin/.

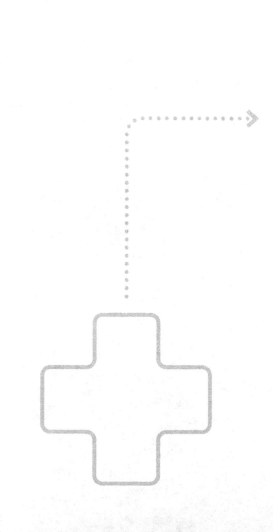

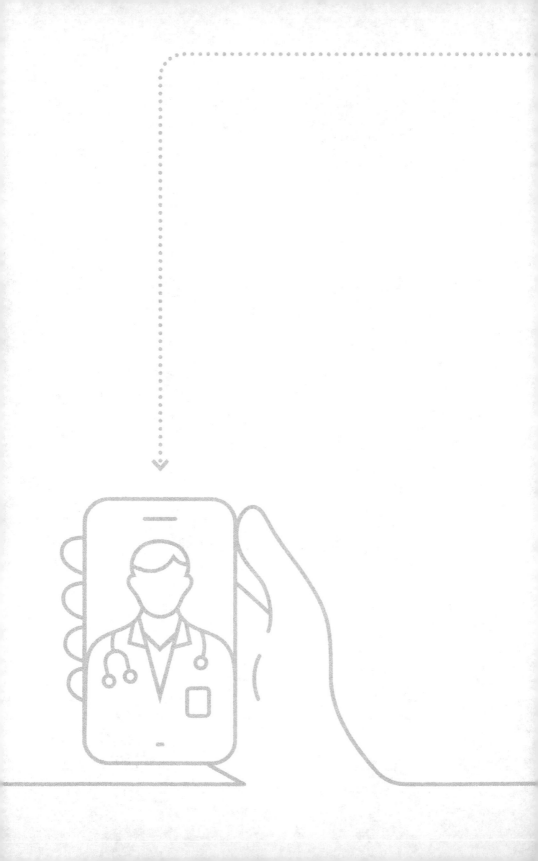

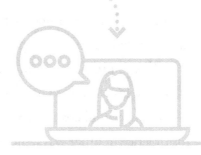

CHAPTER 14

Costs

I n 2018, Michael Heckendorn was a licensed professional counselor practicing outside of Denver. Like most professional counselors, he was renting an office for $750 per month in a shared suite with a number of other therapists, and it was one of his biggest expenses. At first, he added telehealth services to his practice hesitantly, without knowing how many clients would want it. He soon found that offering teletherapy sessions for his adolescent clientele was a wonderful option because busy parents found it hard to get their teens into a physical office each week.

Before long, he was seeing more than half of his clients by video. While a handful of clients still preferred to meet in the office, they weren't numerous enough to justify the cost of rent, so he canceled his lease and signed up at a flex workspace for $10/hour and a $50 monthly membership fee. He also arranged for community-based experiential sessions where he saw patients on nature hikes, at their local climbing gyms, and park pavilions. Teens and families quickly warmed to his new model, which became three teletherapy sessions and one experiential or in-person session per month.

This approach not only saved Michael hundreds of dollars in expenses, but also freed him from having to take on additional clients to cover overhead costs. He spent more time networking and growing his practice in other ways, including hiring additional employees and expanding his network, which increased revenue. When the pandemic hit, he seamlessly transitioned to fully remote and canceled his flex space membership. This chapter focuses on the cost of providing care and will hopefully help you achieve some of the same things that Michael did: cutting costs and maximizing revenue.

Operating Costs

As many found during and after the pandemic, working remotely reduces the need for office space and its associated costs. Medical practices especially stand to benefit, as they spend 60–70 percent on average of their revenue on overhead, including physical space, personnel, medical supplies, and energy. Meanwhile, hospital costs have risen 20 percent since the pandemic, and an astonishing 33 percent of hospitals now operate at a loss.[244] While many of these operational expenses are required for delivery of healthcare, some aren't necessary for telehealth. Anywhere from 20 to 50 percent of clinical operating budgets are spent on real estate alone. [245] In addition to private exam rooms, clinics need a waiting room, office space for staff,

> **Anywhere from 20 to 50 percent of clinical operating budgets are spent on real estate alone.**

space for diagnostic equipment, and storage rooms for medical supplies.

Telehealth also cuts down on variable costs. One study that examined the cost of operating a child psychiatry clinic in rural Kansas compared to telepsychiatry services found that fixed (e.g., office space, admin, insurance, medical records) *and* variable (e.g., salaries, tech support, equipment) costs were significantly higher for in-person care compared to telehealth.[246] Another study on orthopedic consultants in rural Norway found that while telemedicine entailed higher up-front costs, mostly from acquiring telehealth technology, the incremental cost remained lower than in-person care; in effect, telemedicine had a higher cost per person initially but broke even after 183 consultations and became cheaper thereafter.[247] A cost analysis of patients in Australia who received emergency appendectomy or cholecystectomy surgery found that the clinic paid $52.76 per patient for in-person follow up care compared to $19.05 for telehealth follow up care.[248]

Even for clinicians who rotate between in-person and telehealth days, the amount paid in overhead costs, including physical space, energy, and supplies, all go down. When Ethan Bing, the administrator of a multispecialty clinic in Katy, Texas, decided to expand their telehealth options during the pandemic, he found that by making 25 percent of their overall visits virtual, they cut their supply costs by 30 percent.[249] For Ethan, this included "everything from less paper to less table paper sanitizer—it's small stuff, but it adds up." Ethan's clinic was also able to cut staff and hire more part-time employees, which further decreased costs. Telemedicine further allows organizations to get creative by adjusting staff schedules, covering multiple locations, experimenting with utilizing less space, seeing patients off-hours from home, and partnering with outside clinicians.

Telemedicine can also increase the efficiency of healthcare delivery. By allowing clinicians to see more patients in less time, it reduces the need for additional staff to manage patient volumes. When establishing one of the earliest programs of tele-triage at Jefferson, Aditi's team started out using ER doctors to staff their virtual program because they didn't know how patients would react or how well it would work. Once clinical processes were smoothed out, and everyone became familiar with the process and trusted that it was safe, the team gradually switched over to using nurse practitioners and physician assistants. Because of the staffing cost savings, they were able to add another doctor back into their ER, which improved patient flow and efficiency.

With all of this said, healthcare facilities are often obligated to staff a certain level of care. When clinicians are unavailable due to vacation, sick leave, or job transitions, they often turn to *locum tenens* services for temporary staffing, whose associated costs add up. Telemedicine can help reduce costs by decreasing the need for in-person locum tenens by providing them remotely at a reduced rate and adding telehealth services that connect to specialists and other doctors, all of which can reduce staff size.

Telemedicine reduces the need for healthcare providers to travel to remote clinics to see patients, which can decrease travel expenses, including fuel costs, vehicle maintenance, and lodging for healthcare organizations. For instance, a study of telepsychiatrists serving rural Native American populations found that costs were $94 for telehealth compared to $183 for in-person care due to psychiatrists having to travel to remote satellite clinics for in-person appointments. The study also found that the more patients are seen over telehealth, the greater the cost savings and that a multistate center was cheaper than each state operating independently.[250] Similarly, remote retinal evaluations in Hungry saved 92,248 km in transport distances and 3,633 staff working hours, with an annual cost savings ranging from €17,435 to €35,140.[251]

We've already touched on the extent to which telemedicine consistently reduces no-show rates and how much that alone saves organizations. A Canadian study found that reducing even half of their unnecessary missed appointments would save the national healthcare system $58 million annually.[252] When a large federally qualified health center in Texas with twenty-three locations implemented telehealth, it saved $45,578 per month simply from the decreased number of missed appointments. When its support team was proactive about reaching out to patients with upcoming appointment reminders, its savings were even more pronounced.[253]

In the US, unnecessary hospital readmissions cost Medicare approximately $26 billion annually, and in response, CMS no longer reimburses for care provided to patients readmitted within thirty days, along with fines for failing to meet readmission quality metrics—all of which puts hospitals at a huge financial risk. As a result, many hospitals swiftly created new programs using telemedicine to avoid not only readmissions but also incurring the nonreimbursable cost of readmission.[p]

The Cost of Telehealth

There is a cost to starting and running a telehealth program, and it can even be substantial. Telehealth is still a young field, so there's a lot of variability in implementation, which means a wide range of cost. A study that compared telemedicine implementation at nine community health centers in California found that equipment costs made up the

---

p   Covered in chapter 4.

majority of start-up expenses and that the actual cost of equipment also varied significantly. One health center spent over $250,000 on telehealth equipment, where another spent only $3,000.[254] In the same study, total annual operating costs ranged from $137,000 to $1.2 million, which included licenses for vendor software, clinic, and administrative staff.

With the annual volume of telehealth patients ranging from 433 to 7,254, some of these community health centers did not have enough telehealth visits to be profitable. The cost per visit ranged from $67 to $397, and as such, five centers would not break even if they got reimbursed for 100 percent, and one would have needed two thousand more billable patients to reach profitability.

> **If you're not careful, the cost savings of offering telehealth can easily be consumed by operational costs.**

The lesson here is: if you're not careful, the cost savings of offering telehealth can easily be consumed by operational costs, underscoring the importance of basic accounting in setting up your telehealth. It should go without saying that the cost of doing telehealth can't be more than the money your practice generates. The "build-it-and-they-will-come" mentality is not a smart approach. You first need to estimate how many patients you will see, how much that will cost, and how much money you expect to generate or save by using telehealth before you start spending money—especially on equipment.

Ensure what you are purchasing is really what you need, especially when dealing with long-term contracts. You may not need that rolling telemedicine cart with multiple monitors, a PTZ camera, battery backup, and a suite of peripherals that cost as much as a luxury car. A simple, low-cost, software-based solution using your own devices may be all that you need to start. You can also repurpose equipment you already have. When Aditi's team decided to ramp up telehealth in-hospital consults during the pandemic, they repurposed a stack of unused iPads that had been sitting around. Use what's at your disposal, and if you find you truly need to add more features to your telehealth technology, you can always do it later.

We can also say from experience that it's more than likely that you won't. Aditi also spent a good deal of time investigating and then buying a remote stethoscope for virtual visits because she thought she'd still want to hear the lungs and heart virtually during tele-triage. As it turned out, she was wrong; most of her patients were already in the ER so on-site clinical staff took care of it. Nothing was necessarily *wrong* with the digital stethoscope; she simply never used it.

While some costs are fixed or nonnegotiable, contracts for telemedicine equipment, training, and even software licenses fees can be negotiated, especially when they're bought in bulk or entail a long-term commitment. Aditi's team negotiated cheaper rates at Jefferson by offering research contributions, advising on product improvements, referrals, and generally willing to be testers for new products.

Given the costs of real estate, supplies, salaries, and travel, the cost of providing care is expensive. Telemedicine can help healthcare organizations avoid these expenses. To be successful, use telehealth to reduce clinic overhead expenses, make sure your telehealth service doesn't cost more than you can generate, and look for ways to reduce the cost of telehealth, especially in terms of unnecessary equipment.

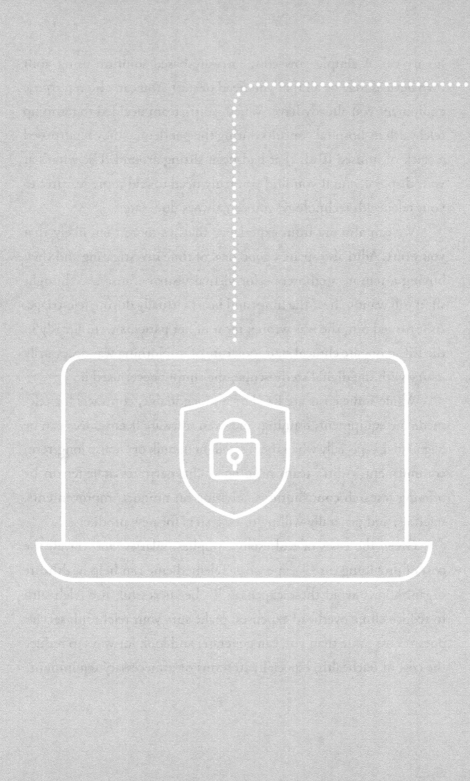

Compliance Success

Brandon M. Welch

H ealthcare is inherently risky, and laws and regulations have been enacted by governing bodies to protect patients from unnecessary harm. Healthcare is also big business and amounts to a staggering $4 trillion annually, or 20 percent of the entire American GDP. The immense amount of money involved attracts a lot of smart and sometimes unscrupulous people. From ordinary people taking advantage of reimbursement policies to hackers holding patient information for ransom, opportunities for exploitation in healthcare are everywhere.

Laws and regulations in healthcare are intended to keep patients safe, ensure their privacy, guard against financial abuse, and promote fairness and equity in healthcare to all. They can be broken down into three types: regulatory, professional, and organizational.

Regulatory laws and regulations are established by governments for the protection and benefit of society. Many, such as malpractice, fraud, and prescribing laws, are in place to protect against harm (chapters 17–19). Others ensure patient privacy rights (chapter 20–22). These are enforced through the judicial system and can result in civil or criminal action, court orders, fines, and even prison sentences for the most serious offenses. As a result, clinicians and health systems generally hire lawyers to deal with the laws around regulations, malpractice, and laws that govern medicine. Regardless, clinicians and administrators will benefit from having a basic working understanding of federal, state, and jurisdictional requirements, if only for their own safety.

Beyond regulatory compliance, professional compliance relates to medical boards, the governing bodies that regulate healthcare (chapter 23). Medical boards are given their authority by governments but act relatively autonomously in presiding over individual states. Professional compliance violations can lead to reprimands, corrective action, or the suspension or revocation of licenses.

Finally, organizational compliance (chapter 24) relates to the internal policies, procedures, and practices dictated by employers. Often, these policies are stricter, established and enforced at the organizational level, and geared toward avoiding professional or regulatory issues. Consequences for not complying with organizational requirements can range from upsetting the boss, to being suspended, to getting fired.

Clinicians must walk a fine line, staying compliant with regulations, but without unnecessarily restricting themselves and the care they provide. All too often, clinicians hinder themselves by following a stricter interpretation of requirements than is necessary, which ultimately makes things harder for them and their patients. It's a delicate balance. If you're overly restrictive, it will impoverish the care experience. Conversely, if you don't adhere to rules and regulations, you could get shut down, or even end up in jail. Most laws and regulations applicable to in-person care tend to automatically apply to telemedicine. However, technology adds an additional layer of risk not present in traditional in-person care, and whether real or perceived, it must be taken into account.

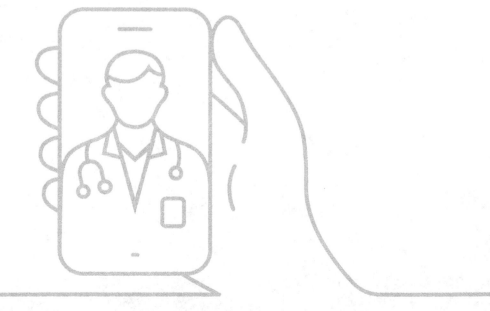

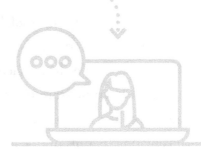

CHAPTER 15

Malpractice

O ne of the most important, precedent-setting cases in the history of telemedicine happened in 2006, back when few people practiced telemedicine or knew about it. A fourteen-year-old named Krystine White, who struggled with mental illness, presented to her clinicians as angry and aggressive and had been cutting herself. Her case manager referred her to a psychiatrist, Mark Harris, MD, with a copy of a recent medical examination that detailed her behavioral issues.

Dr. Harris was located in a different state, so Krystine filled out Dr. Harris's preassessment questionnaire and then participated in a ninety-minute video conference with him. Afterward, Dr. Harris provided Krystine's care team with an evaluation and a description of her illness, offered insight into her problems, and suggested medication and a treatment plan he thought would help. As the services he provided were part of a research protocol, Dr. Harris made it clear he wouldn't be providing follow-up services or prescribing medication.

A year later, Krystine took her own life by overdosing on prescription drugs, and afterward, her family sued Dr. Harris for malpractice. They claimed that he had neglected his duty to exercise reasonable care to protect Krystine from the danger she posed to herself. Dr. Harris countered that he was no longer her clinician beyond their initial consultation, per his protocol.

In the end, the courts decided that even a one-time telemedicine consultation was enough to establish a doctor-patient relationship and that the standard of care required Dr. Harris to follow up. *Standard of care* broadly refers to doing what any other physician with your specific training and experience would reasonably do in the same situation. Examples of deviating from standard of care can be providing unnecessary or inappropriate care, using unconventional treatments, failing to perform a necessary evaluation that would have *led* to a diagnosis, or general negligence on the part of the clinician.

While this was an unexpected and unfortunate outcome for Dr. Harris, this case legally established telemedicine's standard of care as equivalent to in-person care. Since then, from a malpractice perspective, courts have consistently viewed telemedicine sessions between clinicians and patients as meeting standard of care—in other words, it has clinical validity. To be successful with telehealth, it is important to understand that clinicians are legally held to the same standard of care over telehealth as in person.

Do No Harm

Despite the fact that the exact phrase "first, do no harm" doesn't actually exist in the Hippocratic Oath, it's widely accepted as *the* guiding principle in medicine. Harm generally refers to physical pain or death but can include unnecessary suffering, misdiagnosis, hardship, disability, psychological trauma, past or future expenses, and loss of income. Unfortunately, and despite the best of intentions, unnecessary harm can and does still happen, and even unintentional harm can still be considered malpractice.

It's important to remember that harm is a prerequisite for malpractice; if no harm was done, there is no case for malpractice, even if the standard of care was not followed. The harm in question also has to be a direct result of the clinician failing to provide standard of care. Likewise, if harm happened, but the clinician adhered to the standard of care, it's still very hard to make a case for malpractice.

Most of the time there is no *intent* on the part of the clinician to do harm, which is what makes most malpractice cases civil issues. Civil cases, which legally refer to general wrongdoing, are the most common in healthcare. The legal term for these is torts, which broadly refer to loss or harm, breaches of trust, and/or wrongful acts committed against another person or property. The vast majority of civil cases settle outside of court for monetary compensation, which is usually paid by malpractice insurance. Those that don't settle end up in trial. In either case, clinicians are obligated to inform their licensing board about the case. From there, the board may enforce additional penalties, including the suspension of licenses, which can make it harder to get a license in a new state or simply to find a new job.

Malpractice in Telemedicine

Of the estimated twenty thousand medical malpractice lawsuits filed each year in the US, very few cases are related to telemedicine, and even fewer have resulted in trials and judicial decisions. In fact, of all the malpractice cases tried in the US between 2010 and 2022, zero were set in motion by the use of telemedicine, per se; a few happened to *use* telemedicine, but telemedicine itself wasn't the reason for the failure that caused harm.

There are a few likely explanations for this. First, most clinicians use telemedicine for uncomplicated and low-risk patients. Urgent, high-risk cases are mostly handled by in-person care, not telemedicine. Also, the high-risk specialties that see the most malpractice cases, like obstetrics and neurology, are typically sued in direct relation to the in-person care they deliver. Finally, telemedicine usually involves low-dollar-amount clinical cases, so it tends to be less attractive to commission-based litigating attorneys.

> **Many in the industry expect there to be an uptick in malpractice cases involving telemedicine.**

Of course, telemedicine is also quite young in the age of law, and it typically takes several years for a malpractice claim to work its way through the legal system. Given that telemedicine was also a niche concern before Covid, many in the industry expect there to be an uptick in malpractice cases involving telemedicine with time as long as adoption remains high.

When using telemedicine, the first thing to ensure is that you can deliver the same—or at least a similar—level of care, skill, and learning that you would provide in person. Cases that don't require a physical examination, such as counseling, education, or review of results, are similar between in person and telemedicine. A simple audio-video connection is usually sufficient to provide standard of care. The risk of harm is low, so there's not a lot to worry about.

However, for more complicated assessments or treatments that require physical interaction or specialized equipment, achieving the same standard of care between in person and telemedicine may not be possible. For example, one multiple sclerosis study noted the challenge of performing a complete neurologic exam over telehealth.[255] There's still no reliable way for remote neurologists to evaluate tone, sensation, reflexes, and fundoscopy remotely, which collectively pose a risk in terms of misdiagnosis and mismanagement.[256] If a diagnosis could be missed via telemedicine that would have been identified in person, there may be a case for malpractice. If you find that you're unable to provide standard of care via telehealth, it's best to simply see the patient in question in person.

Though very few telemedicine-related malpractice cases have ever occurred, professional liability insurance already has policies in place for when they do. With time, insurance will probably begin to treat telemedicine the same as in-person coverage. Until then, most insurance companies include telemedicine malpractice insurance as a part of their professional liability policies, and others offer it as a separate policy or add-on. It's worth noting that most policies cover claims made only in a specific state, so if you're treating patients in other states, make sure that your policy includes coverage for telemedicine, *and* that your medical liability insurance covers all the states in which you're licensed.

Malpractice is a risk for every provider, and providing care via telehealth presents new risks to providers of all kinds. To be successful with telemedicine, ensure that you're able to provide the same standard of care as in person, and make sure to verify that your professional liability insurance covers telemedicine.

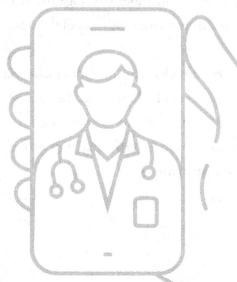

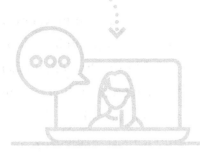

CHAPTER 16

Fraud

One sunny morning in April 2019, dozens of unmarked cars with federal license plates pulled up outside an unassuming office building in Tampa, Florida. Armed Federal Bureau of Investigation (FBI) agents with bulletproof vests quietly entered the building, where they began executing a search-and-seizure warrant of twenty different medical supply companies operating on the premises. For the rest of the day, agents steadily exited the building with confiscated computers and boxes of evidence.

Most of it belonged to Kelly Wolfe, who had been using her medical billing company to falsify documentation and then charge Medicaid for unnecessary orthotic braces, which were sent to elderly beneficiaries who neither needed nor wanted them. All the while, Wolfe had been using the guise of "telemedicine" to explain her company's unusually high volume of claims. Her scheme also involved creating fraudulent orders for brace supplies, using doctors to remotely sign prescriptions for the braces after little to no contact with any of their "patients," submitting claims for reimbursement, and finally giving kickbacks to accomplices through ersatz "telemedicine companies."

Wolfe's $400 million scheme was quelled as part of a nationwide Medicaid fraud crackdown called "Operation Brace Yourself," which resulted in an estimated cost avoidance of more than $1.9 billion for orthotic braces nationally. Wolfe ultimately pleaded guilty, agreed to pay back more than $20 million, and faces up to thirteen years in prison.[257]

Healthcare Fraud

Healthcare fraud has been a problem for as long as modern medicine has existed. Though it comes in many forms, unnecessary costs for unnecessary services are the most common variety. It exists at all levels: patients fake ailments to get a prescription, clinicians upcharge for services they didn't provide, and companies bill for products that aren't medically necessary. Fraud causes tens of billions of dollars in losses each year, compromises the health and safety of patients,

> In 2020 alone, Medicare permanently revoked billing privileges of over 250 medical professionals for their involvement in telemedicine fraud schemes.

and indirectly affects us all though higher insurance premiums and taxes to cover the losses.

Needless to say, committing healthcare fraud is against the law. Those found guilty of fraud are usually required to pay back remunerations for defrauded amounts and fines—and sometimes face prison sentences as well. Any clinician or organization found guilty of committing fraud is prohibited from billing federal healthcare programs for services in perpetuity. In 2020 alone, Medicare permanently revoked billing privileges of over 250 medical professionals for their involvement in telemedicine fraud schemes.[258]

Most healthcare fraud is related to billing. To combat this, the False Claims Act makes it illegal for clinicians or organizations to knowingly submit fraudulent claims to federal health programs, including Medicaid, Medicare, and TRICARE. This includes inflating the time spent providing care, charging excessively, making false statements, billing for services or products that were not medically necessary (or not provided), and claiming greater complexity than reality in order to increase reimbursement.

Telemedicine visits typically entail low-complexity cases, so billing telemedicine service at a higher complexity rate for low-complexity activities is prohibited. Similarly, falsely claiming a telemedicine visit was delivered in person because it generates higher reimbursement is also illegal. Clinicians also should not bill for services that were not provided, even when attempted in good faith; for example, if the telehealth appointment fails to accomplish anything meaningful due to technical issues, the clinician should not seek reimbursement.

Violations of the False Claims Act can result in significant penalties to the clinician or organization, including recovery of three times the amount of the false claim, imprisonment, and an additional penalty of up to $11,000 per claim. Moreover, some states have their own version of the False Claims Act, which can include additional fines and imprisonment. States typically investigate and prosecute false claims against health insurance and private payers, though when insurance fraud spans across several states or federal funding was involved, the FBI will often get involved.

In many industries, it is perfectly acceptable to compensate those who refer business to you, but it's illegal for government-funded healthcare programs such as Medicare. Kickbacks create a noncompetitive service delivery, which potentially leads to overutilization and increased costs of healthcare services. In turn, the Federal Anti-Kickback Statute prohibits the use of remuneration to induce referrals for any product or services paid for by government-funded healthcare programs. In addition to financial remuneration, prohibited kickbacks can include free or very low rent for office space and excessive compensation for medical directorships.q Those who pay or accept kickbacks also face penalties of up to $50,000 plus three times the amount of the kickback *and* up to five years in prison. To compound the issue, if the claim came from a kickback, it may be considered a fraudulent claim and thus a violation of the False Claims Act.

Similarly, the Stark Laws are civil laws that prohibit a physician from referring patients to an entity with which they, or an immediate family member, have a financial relationship. Penalties include denial of payment, refund of reimbursement received, and penalties of up to $15,000.

In spite of all of the above, conspirators still seek ways to conceal illegal kickbacks and bribes. Fraudsters often make payments indirectly through shell companies via bank accounts located both inside and outside of the US and then hide their companies' existence through false statements to financial institutions and the IRS. In addition to facing serious prison time for healthcare fraud and kickbacks, these

---

q   Both Anti-Kickback Statute and Stark Laws have exemptions, called "safe harbor" regulations, that allow specific payment or business practices to exist that would otherwise trigger a violation. https://oig.hhs.gov/compliance/safe-harbor-regulations/.

schemes also entail five additional years for each count of tax evasion and twenty additional years for money laundering.

Telemedicine Fraud

Fraud involving so-called telemedicine is currently on the rise, largely because it's relatively quick and easy for criminals to commit crimes on a vast scale. In 2020, $4.5 billion of the $6 billion-plus in overall fraud losses were due to telemedicine schemes.[259] In the aforementioned National Health Care Fraud Takedown alone, over eighty criminal defendants in nineteen judicial districts were arrested for false and fraudulent claims involving telemedicine, and over 250 medical professionals were punished for their involvement.

It's hard for a single individual to commit fraud on that scale. A "successful" scheme will usually involve multiple players working together to evade regulations and oversight. The most common telemedicine fraud schemes proceed in a similar fashion. The owners of telemarketing companies are typically the masterminds behind the schemes. First, these individuals will rebrand a traditional telemarketing call center as a "telemedicine company." Next, call center employees contact a list of Medicare beneficiaries offering a "free" product or service, such as orthotic braces, genetic tests, or medicated creams. The employee then confirms that the patient is eligible to receive benefits, collects their pertinent health information, and creates an order on the patient's behalf—sometimes with and sometimes without their knowledge.

Next, the company pays kickbacks, bribes, or salaries to a licensed healthcare professional to review and sign the prefilled orders, typically after little to no interaction with the "patient." Medical equipment companies, laboratories, or pharmacies then purchase batches of signed orders from the company, which are subsequently billed to Medicare. To make these schemes work, conspirators pay kickbacks indirectly using shell companies and bank accounts in and out of the US. Sadly, at some point, each and every variation on the telemedicine fraud scheme described above involves a licensed clinician.

Here it's important to reiterate that healthcare in the US is a trust-based system in which licensed healthcare clinicians play a central role, and medical licensing sets a high bar to ensure that clinicians are trained, qualified, and honest. In exchange for this trust and authority, clinicians are expected to abide by relevant laws and regulations and to be a backstop against fraudsters. Because payers, suppliers, pharmacies, and laboratories rely on clinician signatures to confirm that a product or service is medically needed, fraudsters need a clinician's prescribing authority to commit fraud in the first place.

Given their gatekeeping role, if clinicians violate this trust, they will ultimately be held accountable and liable for far more than they ever stood to benefit from fraud schemes. Yet most clinicians are not trying to be malicious; many are just moonlighting as subcontractors and wholly unaware that they're participating in fraud. Licensed healthcare clinicians are usually just pawns to the fraudsters, often earning a paltry $20–$30 per prescription while the real criminals rake in millions of dollars. Yet, because of their gatekeeping role as licensed clinicians, they remain liable for losses entailed, which often far exceed whatever they made from their participation in a broader scheme. Even if the clinician didn't know they were part of a fraud scheme, if they failed to follow policies or guidelines that would have prevented the fraud, then they can be held liable, lose billing privileges, and face administrative action, fines, and/or prison time.

Bernard Ogon, MD is a good example. He received a thirty-three-month prison sentence and was ordered to pay restitution of

$24.3 million for his role enabling a telemedicine fraud scheme to prescribe expensive compounded medications. A "telemedicine" company had been sending him prefilled prescription forms to sign, with little or no information about the patients in question. The telemedicine companies paid Ogon $20–$30 for each prescription he signed, yet the fraud caused losses of over $20 million.[260]

In another scheme, a nurse practitioner, Richard Laksonen, signed batches of prewritten orders for knee braces. By signing, he attested that he had performed the assessments and had verified that the orders were reasonable and medically necessary. In reality, he signed orders without reviewing the records and spent eighteen seconds on average per order. In a one-week period, Lacksonen signed over three hundred. He ultimately pleaded guilty to making a false statement related to healthcare matters and was subsequently sentenced to twenty-one months in federal prison followed by three years of supervised release. In addition, he was ordered to pay $6 million in restitution to Medicare.[261]

Under the False Claims Act, there does not need to be an intent to defraud. "Deliberate ignorance" or "reckless disregard" is sufficient to convict. Even if a clinician is oblivious to the larger web they're a part of, they can still be held fully liable for their part in failing to prevent fraud. Dr. Le Thu, an emergency medicine physician, was told that nurses had already consulted with her patients, taken their medical histories, and determined that compounded medication or medical equipment was medically appropriate. She was paid $35 to sign orders, despite never speaking to patients or establishing a clinician-patient relationship.[262] In reality, her "nurses" were located in the Philippines, were not registered to practice in the US, and had never spoken with the patients in question. Dr. Thu was charged with conspiracy to commit healthcare fraud and conspiracy to violate the federal Anti-Kickback Statute, punishable by a fine of $250,000 and up to five years in prison.

Fighting Telemedicine Fraud

Over the past several years, many in the telemedicine industry have advocated for less regulation, making it easier for telemedicine services to provide greater convenience, value, and benefit to patients, clinicians, and the healthcare system as a whole. At the same time, lifting these regulations can also make it easier for criminals to abuse the system. People who take advantage of telehealth to commit fraud are harming the industry because fraud gives a bad name to the broader telemedicine industry. When a major healthcare fraud is announced involving a shady, unaccredited "telemedicine" company, it erodes public trust for legitimate telemedicine companies, services, and clinicians in general.

While clinicians tend to enjoy the highest trust across industries, announcements of major fraud involving complicit doctors negatively impacts trust across healthcare. If excessive abuse and harm continue, additional regulations and laws will be necessary to protect against them. The bigger the problem, the more restrictive the regulations and rules will become, all of which will make it harder for law-abiding clinicians to provide care to patients who could benefit the most from it.

Because the federal government is the largest payer of healthcare in the US, they see the greatest amount of fraud and direct the most resources toward fighting it. This job mostly falls upon the Health Care Fraud Strike Force, an interagency team made up of investigators and prosecutors including the FBI, the Department of Justice (DOJ), and the Department of Health and Human Services' Office of Inspector General (HHS-OIG). In all, sixteen strike forces operate in twenty-seven districts to prevent and deter fraud.

To target and take down perpetrators, they rely on traditional investigative techniques as well as advanced data analysis to identify suspicious billing patterns. Fortunately for honest telemedicine clinicians, the Strike Force maintains a positive perspective of telemedicine; its goal is "ensuring that telehealth delivers quality, convenient care for patients, and is not compromised by fraud." As the Strike Forces enforces antifraud laws, the HHS-OIG focuses on preventing healthcare waste, fraud, and abuse. They're responsible for advising policymakers and stakeholders, and they regularly put out special fraud alerts about telemedicine schemes, as well as guides for clinicians on how to avoid being caught up in fraud schemes.[263]

MedPac, another nonpartisan independent legislative branch agency, provides Congress with analysis and policy advice on Medicaid and Medicare. To prevent telehealth fraud, they recommended additional scrutiny to outlier clinicians who prescribe or bill more than their peers, and generally require clinicians to have a face-to-face visit before ordering high-cost medical equipment or clinical lab tests. The Telehealth Extension Act, which aims to make permanent many of the telemedicine restrictions that were lifted during the Covid public health emergency, includes the MedPac recommendations.

Despite broad government efforts to stamp out telemedicine fraud, it's impossible for regulators to catch everything. Fraud at any level is harmful to the healthcare industry and needs to be stopped—period. It's incumbent upon clinicians, administrators, executives, and even patients to ensure the integrity of the healthcare system by fighting fraud.

Understanding what is and is not permissible is the first and most important step in avoiding fraud. As such, healthcare organizations should maintain a strong culture of compliance, which includes training, prevention, and detection of activities that do not adhere to laws and guidelines. If you see something, say something. Since many fraud schemes require a licensed healthcare professional's signature, clinicians are in an excellent position to either enable *or* deter fraud schemes. If you see, are approached by, or suspect someone in violating a law or regulation, don't look the other way. It's your duty to notify authorities.

> **Being a whistleblower can often be more financially rewarding than participating in fraud itself.**

Fortunately, antifraud laws include provisions that protect and incentivize those who do the right thing. The False Claims Act notably protects whistleblowers from discrimination, harassment, suspension, or termination of employment as a result of reporting possible fraud. Being a whistleblower can often be more financially rewarding than participating in fraud itself; individuals who report fraud may be entitled to receive 15–25 percent of the government's recovery if they file a lawsuit on behalf of the US. A former employee of Kelly Wolfe will receive 23 percent of the $20.3 million civil recovery as her reward for notifying the feds about her fraud scheme. If you have been involved with or suspect a fraudulent telemedicine scheme, contact the FBI hotline at 1-800-CALL-FBI.

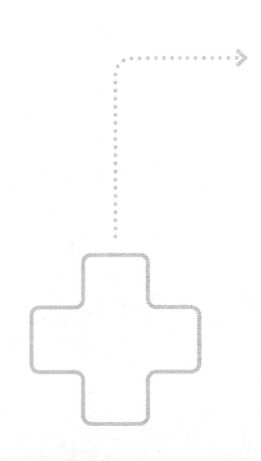

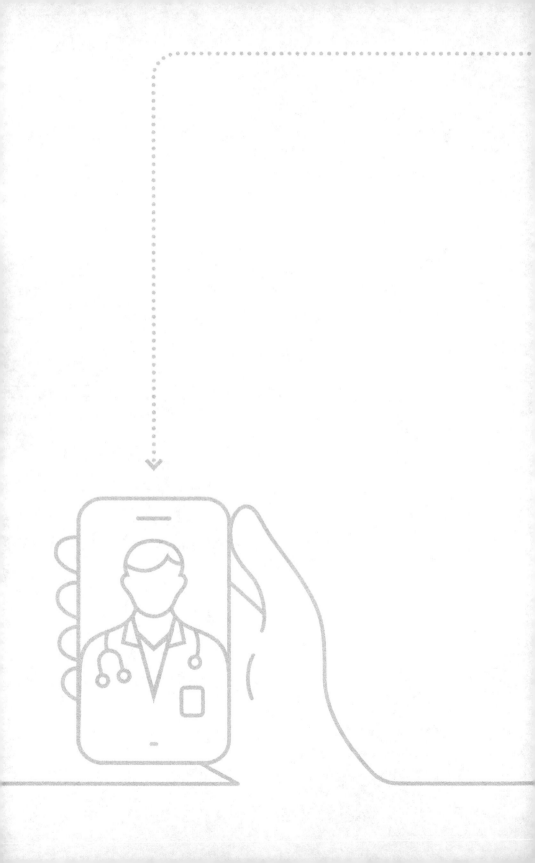

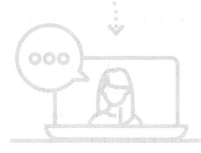

CHAPTER 17

Prescribing Laws

H umans have always used natural substances for healing, and as soon as remedies were first sold directly to consumers, unscrupulous actors appeared to take advantage of the desperate. With the rise of scientific medicine in the late nineteenth century, governments began to regulate and protect the public from misuse, abuse, and dependence on harmful substances. Ever since, prescribing laws have shaped the industry of medicine, including telemedicine, both for better and for worse. To be successful with telemedicine, it is important to know applicable prescribing rules and regulations because prescribing certain drugs in certain situations via telemedicine may violate applicable laws.

Controlled Substances

In response to the rise in use and abuse of barbiturates and amphetamines in the mid-twentieth century, the Controlled Substances Act was passed in 1970. This law brought all drugs with abuse potential under the purview of the Drug Enforcement Agency (DEA) and defined the five schedules to classify them based upon their potential for physical or mental dependence, abuse, medical utility, and safety. Controlled substances are the most heavily regulated medications and can be prescribed only for a legitimate medical purpose during the course of clinical care.[264]

Schedule I drugs like heroin or cocaine have high abuse potential and no accepted medical use, so physicians are prohibited from prescribing them altogether. Schedule II drugs like oxycodone have an accepted medical use *and* a high potential for abuse. Given their high potential for addiction, these drugs are subject to higher regulation and oversight. Schedule III, IV, and V drugs have progressively lower potential for abuse and have acceptable medical use in treatment.

Physicians generally have the highest prescriptive authority and are authorized to prescribe Schedule II drugs with a valid Drug Enforcement Administration (DEA) license. Some states also allow nurse practitioners and physician's assistants to prescribe Schedule II drugs, although these come with additional requirements, including training, certificates, and/or physician oversight. While there's technically no limit to the amount of controlled substances a clinician can prescribe, some states have implemented additional regulations and oversight.

The Controlled Substance Act provided enough protection to patients for the better part of two decades, but then the internet came along, and one notable case highlights the challenges of the era. In 2001, eighteen-year-old Ryan Haight, an honor student from La Mesa, California, was found lying unconscious in his bedroom from an accidental drug overdose. His death was the result of a combination of narcotics that had been legally prescribed, purchased, and dispensed from an out-of-state prescriber and online pharmacy.

Though both of Ryan's parents were healthcare professionals and well aware of the dangers in using controlled substances, he'd been covertly experimenting with his medications without their knowledge. Ryan wasn't an isolated case. In the early 2000s, the proliferation of rogue online pharmacies selling controlled substances directly to patients online with little to no oversight was wreaking havoc on thousands of Americans.

In hopes of preventing similar tragedies from ever happening again, in 2008 Congress passed the Ryan Haight Act, which requires clinicians to conduct at least one in-person medical evaluation before prescribing any controlled substance and prevents physicians from signing prescriptions for patients en masse without an established clinician-patient relationship. The act shut down an entire industry of rogue pharmacies and prescribers and continues to protect people from illicit abuse of controlled substances today.

However, one of the law's unfortunate side effects has been to make it more challenging for ethical clinicians to legitimately prescribe and dispense controlled substances through telemedicine. In the intervening years, the act's in-person requirement has become a superficial indicator for true clinician-patient relationships.[r] Covid highlighted the barriers created by the rules and the DEA, and a broad acknowledgement of the need for change in prescribing laws for telemedicine followed. In response, the DEA has since proposed rule changes that will require an initial in-person exam before any prescription can be

---

r   There are exceptions to the in-person requirement, including when a public health emergency has been declared. Patients in the care of a DEA-registered facility or clinician, Indian Health Services, and the VA are also exempt. Of course, clinicians must continue to comply with the laws and regulations of the state in which they are practicing.

issued via telemedicine for Schedule II medication or a Schedule III to V narcotic medication.[s]

State Prescribing Regulations

While the federal government sets the baseline for prescribing regulations, it largely relies on state medical boards to govern and enforce their laws, and states have the right to further extend those laws as they see fit. Some states require clinicians to complete additional registrations to prescribe controlled substances or enroll in state-run prescription drug monitoring programs. Others take a more reactionary approach, monitoring for unusual prescribing patterns or waiting for complaints to commence action. States can also add medications that require prescriptions to controlled-substance schedules, making them even more restrictive than the Ryan Haight Act.

Sometimes, these additional state regulations impede medical practice. For example, in 2019, a university psychiatrist at a large undergraduate institution moved away for another job opportunity, and the university had a hard time finding a replacement to serve its twenty-one thousand students. It eventually turned to Dr. Chris Pelic, a psychiatrist and professor at MUSC, four hours away in Charleston. Dr. Pelic was already using telemedicine with his own patients, so doing the same for these students was a natural fit. For a time, Dr. Pelic, the university, and the students were all safe and happy with his tele-psychiatry services. However, there were federal and state rules that impacted his practice.

Several psychiatric medications are controlled substances, and, ultimately, Dr. Pelic ran into challenges related to their use with telemedicine in treating attention-deficit hyperactivity disorder (ADHD)

---

s   With the exception of buprenorphine.

and anxiety. In South Carolina, Schedule II medications are not to be prescribed via telemedicine unless otherwise approved by the medical board. Given that there was not an available in-person psychiatrist, scope of care for the students was impacted for a period.

As Dr. Pelic requested a waiver for Schedule II medications from the state medical board. When it was denied, he had to travel to the state capital in Columbia to plead his case before the board. There, he met a board of late-career doctors who were initially suspicious of his intentions and concerned for the safety and welfare of his patients. He successfully made the argument that leaving students without a prescribing psychiatrist would ultimately cause far more harm than prescribing antidepressants over video.

In another case of a well-meaning law causing more harm than good, Alabama also passed a law prohibiting clinicians from prescribing controlled substances via telemedicine without an in-person encounter. As a result of this law, Bicycle Health, a California-based telemedicine service who had been treating patients nationwide for opioid use disorder, had to inform its Alabama patients of its obligation to transition to local clinicians for care.[265]

Then, less than a month before the deadline, only 20 percent of their patients were able to find one. To avoid a mass discontinuation of care for these vulnerable patients, Bicycle Health orchestrated what came to be called the "Alabama Airdrop." The company flew two Alabama-licensed physicians to Birmingham, where they met with nearly three hundred patients in a hotel conference room over three days. The law that intended to protect patients effectively created an artificial shortage; Bicycle Health no longer treats new patients in Alabama because of this law.

States can also implement regulations that extend beyond controlled substances. For instance, when the FDA loosened rules related to the home use of abortion medications mifepristone and misoprostol and removed the requirement for in-person dispensing, several abortion clinics began to ramp up their telehealth services. In response, several states proposed bills that would reinstate the old FDA rules.[266] Now there is a state-by-state patchwork of rules regarding prescribing abortion medication over telehealth. As of 2023, more than half of states have passed laws requiring at least one in-person visit before receiving medication for abortion, with some states explicitly banning the use of telemedicine to receive abortion medication.[267] As the Supreme Court overturned Roe v. Wade in 2022, the issue of abortion rights is again returning to the states, and additional telehealth restrictions are likely to follow.

> **Many well-intentioned clinicians remain unaware of the rules, while others don't consider breaking them "a big deal."**

Fortunately, the Ryan Haight Act does not limit the prescription of the noncontrolled substances that account for 90 percent of pharmaceuticals. Treatment for infections and chronic disease, antibiotics, antifungal medications, remedies for blood pressure, insulin, and asthma inhalers are all noncontrolled substances that can be prescribed over telemedicine. Because over-the-counter medications and prescriptions for medical devices and supplies are also considered noncontrolled and aren't bound by the same in-person prescribing requirements, some direct-to-consumer telemedicine companies can offer their services completely online. Companies such as Hims and GetRoman, which offer treatment for men's health issues like hair loss and erectile dysfunction, typically do not deal with controlled substances—so they aren't typically constrained by the in-person rule prior to prescribing. However, some states do have more restrictive prescribing laws that extend beyond controlled substances. For instance, erectile dysfunction medication is not available through online services in South Carolina or North Dakota, and prescribing dermatology products online is prohibited in Louisiana.[268]

With so many different state prescribing requirements, it's easy to be confused by all the different rules. Many well-intentioned clinicians remain unaware of the rules, while others don't consider breaking them "a big deal." Don't be one of these clinicians. Because clinicians are ultimately those deemed responsible if and when something goes wrong, you could be exposed to legal liability.

A Covid Boon Creates a Bust

As emergency waivers eased prepandemic barriers like the Ryan Haight Act, the situation enabled certain services to flourish. Perhaps the most famous of these was Cerebral, which provided prescriptions for controlled substances for a wide range of behavioral health conditions like ADHD, anxiety, depression, and more.

Cerebral's initial launch came one month before the start of Covid, and as the pandemic raged on, it dramatically expanded access to care. After two years, it facilitated 1.8 million visits for over four hundred thousand patients. Its exceptional growth made them the darlings of the investment community, and the future looked bright. Then, a few employee whistleblowers claimed that the company was not conducting visits appropriate to standard of care, called attention to fake accounts seeking illicit prescriptions for resale on the black market, and alleged that the company was prioritizing increasing prescription orders instead of cracking down. Even Cerebral patients themselves raised concerns as many received prescriptions for Adderall or Xanax after brief assessments with minimal follow-up.

In early 2022, Cerebral came under investigation by the Department of Justice for potential violations of controlled substance laws. In response, the company ceased all activities related to controlled substance prescriptions and fired its founder and CEO. In his place, the company promoted its chief medical officer, the Harvard-trained psychiatrist David Mau, to take the helm. Dr. Mau has since renewed focus on training clinicians to adhere to the most up-to-date clinical guidelines. As the government continues to recognize the extent to which patients have relied on greater access to care that telemedicine offers, Cerebral's story has made it wary of the pitfalls of relaxing the rules. Moving forward in this environment will continue to be a delicate tightrope walk, but wherever the law ends up, it's essential to follow appropriate safeguards against harm and abuse.

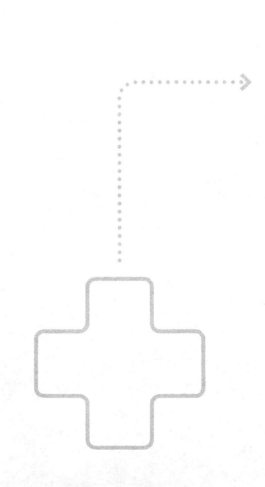

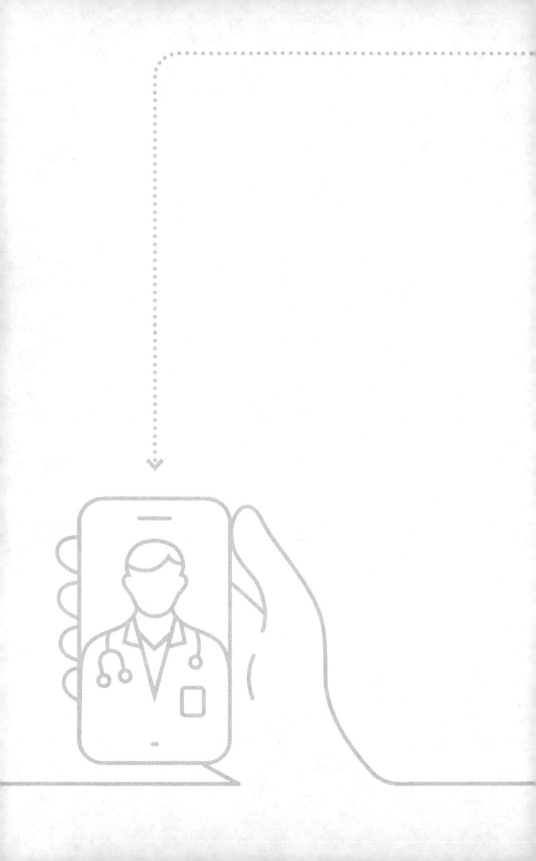

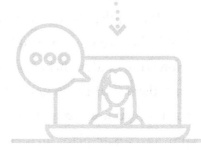

CHAPTER 18

Patient Privacy

When Dion Rambo founded Telehealth Vans at the start of Covid, his goal was to provide an effective way for clinicians from the Los Angeles Department of Mental Health, Probation, and Social Services to meet with the hard-to-reach, low-income, and homeless clients in the area. His concept was simple: he would send out a van equipped with a computer, large monitor, camera, speakers, and mobile internet to facilitate telehealth calls with patients where *they* were located.[t]

In the beginning, Dion thought his team were simply providing a conduit between agency clinicians and their clients. But what made Telehealth Vans even more popular among its vulnerable patients was simply providing a safe, private space for patients to meet with their clinicians. Some patients were homeless women who were forced to live with violent men for shelter, and others were children in unhealthy foster care situations that often lead to jail or prostitution.

---

t   https://doxy.me/en/resources/podcasts/
     ep-12-delivering-telehealth-to-your-door-with-the-telehealth-van-and-dion-rambo/.

Previously, clients were caught in a difficult situation: on one hand, they were often unable to travel to clinics where they could express the need for help, and on the other, when agency workers met with them in their homes, they were unable to ask for help because their perpetrator was present or nearby. Dion discovered that the vans provided a safe place for victims of domestic violence to step away from their unsafe environments—a place to say, "Please, help get me out of here." The ability to seek and receive help was made possible largely because their privacy was assured.

Privacy in Healthcare

Privacy is a fundamental right. In various ways, privacy is guaranteed by the Bill of Rights, which covers the privacy of beliefs and thoughts, personal property, unreasonable searches, and personal information that could lead to self-incrimination.[u] Most breaches of privacy are benign, but some can lead to embarrassment, stigma, discrimination, financial harm, or the tainting of one's reputation and dignity.

Privacy is also a *societal* norm; the perceptions and expectations of privacy among individuals and groups vary. What may be considered intensely private by one person may not be by another. As a result, various states and nations of the world often have differing privacy laws and regulations. In the US, most privacy laws go back to the 1970s, when personal information held in government, school, and bank records started to become digitized. In the 1980s, further laws were passed to protect against intrusive searches using electronic surveillance, wiretapping, and unauthorized access to telephones and computers.

The Health Insurance Portability and Accountability Act (HIPAA) was passed in 1996 to extend privacy protections into

---

u   See the First, Third, Fourth, and Fifth Amendments respectively.

healthcare. While HIPAA remains widely recognized as *the* law in protecting the privacy of patient health information, that wasn't its original intent. It was originally created to help employees maintain health insurance when losing or changing jobs and to simplify the administration of health insurance by standardizing the information shared between health plans, billing services, and healthcare clinicians. Yet ever since, HIPAA has become synonymous with healthcare privacy, mostly because it was the first law that included provisions for privacy in healthcare.

Since then, additional rules, laws, and extensions have gradually filled in privacy gaps and cleared up gray areas. The most notable of these was the Health Information Technology for Economic and Clinical Health (HITECH) Act, which was passed as part of the 2009 Federal Economic Recovery Package. It set rules to further protect the privacy of digital patient information and incentivized healthcare organizations to digitally maintain that information.

Simply understanding a few things about privacy will allow your team to move forward with confidence.

There's often a bit of uncertainty and fear around breaking privacy laws and facing harsh consequences, which often leads to overreaction or avoidance. While high-profile violations have certainly occurred, they're not a huge threat for most providers. Simply understanding a few things about privacy will allow your team to move forward with confidence. When most people talk about privacy, they're often referring to informational privacy, but physical privacy is even more foundational and can't be overlooked.[v]

---

v   See chapter 20.

Physical Privacy

Physical privacy refers to freedom from contact with other people, the desire to limit physical accessibility, and the ability to maintain one's own physical space. Unwelcome physical intrusion, being observed or watched by others, or unwanted contact by another person are all infringements of physical privacy. Common law-enforcement practices like searches, surveillance, and checkpoints all amount to invasions of physical privacy and are the cause for much debate.

Few other industries require individuals to sacrifice physical privacy to the extent of healthcare. Probing questions, physical observation, touching, and in some cases nudity are necessary and accepted aspects of proper clinical examination and treatment. In turn, patients expect their clinicians to protect against unnecessary exposure. Unauthorized physical observations, conversation within earshot of other patients, keeping a door open during medical discussions, or the presence of nonessential medical attendants, spectators, or cameras in the clinic are all common invasions of physical privacy.[w] All of these examples extend to telemedicine, which has its own additional considerations to consider while providing remote care; these include where the patient and clinician are located and how access to virtual meeting rooms are managed.

PATIENT LOCATION

When a user of Doxy.me remarked how well video calls worked even while one of her clients was riding the New York City subway, I was less concerned with the reliability of our service and more surprised that anyone would be comfortable having a call with their doctor

---

w   In teaching hospitals, medical students who are involved in patient care are not considered to be "unwanted observers."

on a busy subway. Yet patients have a surprisingly wide range of tolerance for privacy while on telemedicine calls; some don't think twice about discussing their antidepressant regimen with a clinician from a crowded coffee shop, while others are only comfortable from the quiet privacy of their cars.

While home tends to be the most private place for patients to meet with their clinicians, it's not always the case. For instance, one therapist found it unusual that his patient was always driving during his appointments. After several sessions, the therapist finally brought it up. The patient replied that he didn't want his wife to know he was meeting with a therapist. Since she was tracking his location, he had to act like he was running errands to avoid arousing his wife's suspicion. Similarly, one study found that HIV-positive women cited lack of privacy as their main reason for declining to conduct video counseling sessions at home; 70 percent had not disclosed their HIV status and were concerned about family members overhearing their sessions.[269, 270]

As telemedicine has made it easier for patients to meet with clinicians without taking time off of work, patients also seek privacy wherever they are located. For instance, many patients schedule tele-health sessions on their lunch breaks to meet from the privacy of their cars or reserve private meeting rooms at their offices so coworkers don't overhear their conversations.

It's important to never assume that a given environment is private, even if it appears to be. Clinical staff in a VA clinic in South Dakota inadvertently placed two patients in the same room for their video appointments, instead of two separate rooms. A remote clinician then conducted the video session with the first patient, all without knowing of the second patient's presence until the very end of the call.[271] During the visit, the first patient's name and medical information were discussed in front of the second patient; to avoid similar situations and protect patient privacy while on video calls, have patients confirm that they're alone and in a satisfactory, comfortable, and private location.

CLINICIAN LOCATION

While telehealth affords clinicians the flexibility to provide care wherever they are, they must remain cognizant of their own environments at all times. Clinicians must take reasonable steps to prevent others from overhearing conversations to prevent accidental disclosure. It's best to conduct video calls in a private room with the door shut. It's also prudent to use headphones while speaking in a lowered voice. Whether in the home or a clinic setting, the space should be private and distraction free.

> **Needless to say, clinicians should avoid scheduling and conducting telemedicine calls in public locations.**

Needless to say, clinicians should avoid scheduling and conducting telemedicine calls in public locations. We've heard of clinicians conducting telemedicine calls and discussing private patient information from cafes, which is clearly unprofessional. On the other hand, if an urgent call comes in while you're in a public place, privacy might not be possible; just do your best to limit the identifiable information that's spoken out loud. In such situations, the HIPAA Privacy Rule does allow for limited incidental disclosures to occur that cannot reasonably be prevented.

TELEMEDICINE ACCESS

The last aspect of "physical" privacy in telemedicine concerns access to the online room where virtual interactions happen because a number of scenarios can compromise physical privacy. Perhaps the most well-known is "Zoombombing," where unauthorized parties join and disrupt Zoom meetings, which became popular during Covid. Most virtual access breaches, however, are accidental and not malicious—the digital equivalent of walking into an unlocked occupied clinic room during an in-person appointment. Yet when equipment technicians or other patients accidentally log into an active telehealth session with a patient, this is still considered a breach.[272] This was a more common occurrence with older telemedicine technology but can still happen with more modern technology today.

To prevent unauthorized individuals from joining a telemedicine call, clinicians should use reasonable safeguards. The most important and effective is to simply not give patients the ability to initiate or join calls uninvited. Use telemedicine solutions that give clinicians control over access, including virtual waiting rooms, patient queues, login and passwords, passcodes, and/or unique time-limited meeting invite URLs.

Another form of access privacy is related to the identity of the patient. Most telehealth patients establish their clinician-patient relationships in person, but telemedicine enables these relationships to be established entirely online. This can create situations in which a clinician can mistake Patient A for Patient B and then inadvertently disclose private information about another patient. The risk for identity fraud also increases here because people can more easily claim they're someone they're not virtually than in person.

To avoid these kinds of privacy breaches, clinicians should verify the identity of their patients up front, preferably by verifying the patient's identification over video. A second strategy is to confirm two or more pieces of identifying information, whether that's a patient's social security number, birthday, or middle name. Similarly, clinicians themselves should also identify themselves and the purpose of the visit at the start of the call, which helps to verify that patients are in the right place, at the right time, for the right reason.

Lastly, a breach of physical privacy can also happen by association. For example, showing up at an HIV clinic can implicate an individual being HIV-positive simply by their presence on the premises. As a result, HIV clinics are encouraged to be discreet in their naming to protect their patients' privacy. Similar principles can apply to telehealth. Leaving digital footprints behind on shared computers, whether through URLs, downloadable apps, or saved form field information can lead to indirect privacy disclosure by inference. It's unlikely this could cause a *serious* breach yet remains something to consider in how we design and use telehealth.

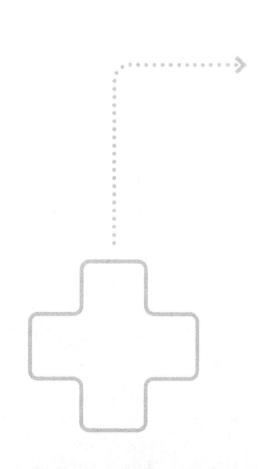

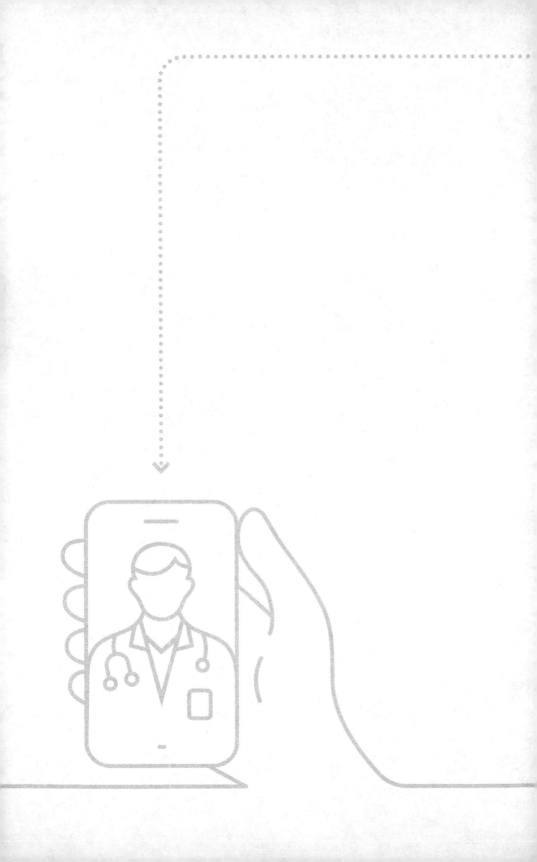

CHAPTER 19

Information Privacy

W e can't provide comprehensive healthcare without collecting information from patients; doing so is necessary to provide the requisite care, make diagnoses, create treatment plans, and provide information for documentation and billing. But this free flow of patient information needs to be balanced with protections to keep information private and confidential. When paper records were the only way to store patient data, it was relatively easy to protect filing cabinets, paper copies, and faxes from unauthorized access, but electronic information is not limited by time and space. As healthcare has become digitized, private health information can instantly travel great distances, and it persists indefinitely. As such, additional care must be taken to prevent unauthorized access and ensure that digital health information stays private.

Dozens of data privacy laws around the world, including HIPAA (US) and the GDPR (EU), have been designed to protect the privacy of electronic information. Many states, including California, are even starting to pass their own data privacy laws. These laws tend to follow the same fundamental principles: limiting the information that is collected, securing it, and building in accountability for failures. We won't get into all the specifics of each law here, but we will explain fundamental principles so you can broadly adhere to them. As you learn these requirements and evaluate your telehealth options, it's particularly worth considering whether storing your patients' information persistently is worth the additional effort and liability.

Transient versus Persistent Data

Before ensuring that your patient's information is private, first seek to understand whether patient information is even being collected and stored; though patient information may be flowing through a technology product, it doesn't necessarily mean it's being *saved* there. For example, an electronic weight scale may create digital information about a patient, but if it doesn't store and associate that data with an individual, it doesn't need to be HIPAA-compliant.

> **Though patient information may be flowing through a technology product, it doesn't necessarily mean it's being *saved* there.**

HIPAA has a notable "conduit exception." When sending physical medical records through the USPS, neither the postman nor the post office needs to be HIPAA compliant. Though the post office is "handling" patient health information, it is considered merely a transient *conduit* of information.[x] Similarly, internet and telephone vendors that solely transfer digital data without storing it are also considered transient conduits and thus are HIPAA-exempt.

---

x   It's a federal crime to open a stamped envelope intended for someone else.

This conduit exception is limited to transmission-only services—once information is stored and becomes persistent within that application or service, *then* HIPAA requirements apply. And while some telehealth solutions don't store patient information and simply act as a conduit, they're still expected to be HIPAA-compliant. This is because the telemedicine software is also involved in the creation and presentation of information in addition to transferring it.

Acting as a conduit and *not* storing patient information persistently is the most secure approach to information privacy. After all, when you don't store patient information persistently, there's nothing that can be compromised. This is the approach video conferencing services like Zoom and Doxy.me take. Because patients don't create accounts, no identifiable patient information is stored. To these systems, patients are essentially anonymous. The audio and video of the call exists only in the moment (as long as the session isn't being recorded). Because files, documents, and messages that contain patient information that is exchanged during the session are not stored when a given session ends, no persistent record exists, significantly reducing the risk of an information breach.

However, even when a service doesn't store patient information, there are still vulnerabilities to consider if the transient information in question isn't adequately protected. This is why Zoom was hit with a class action lawsuit in 2020 for falsely claiming to use "end-to-end encryption."[273] At the time, Zoom used an intermediary server that decrypted video from the sender during transmission and then reencrypted it before sending it on to the receiver. This wasn't true "end-to-end" encryption because the intermediary decryption created a vulnerability that could have allowed a bad actor to access the transient information. Fortunately, there are no known cases where a patient's transient information was exposed, and Zoom has used encrypted intermediary servers ever since.

Identifiability and Sensitivity

As soon as patient information is stored, additional protections become necessary. The more information you store, the higher the obligation and risk you run in keeping it secure. Something as simple as requiring a patient to create an account and log in creates identifiable information, even if nothing else is stored. What constitutes identifiable information under one law may be different under another. Some data privacy laws, including HIPAA, explicitly define eighteen types of information that are considered identifiable. Others, including the General Data Protection Regulation (GDPR), do not define identifiable data in a prescriptive way, and rely instead on *principles*, as in "data can be used to identify someone."

> **The best and easiest approach is to simply *protect all identifiable information*.**

Regardless of what law you're obligated to follow, the best and easiest approach is to simply *protect all identifiable information*. Any information that can be used to distinguish or personally identify an individual is identifiable information and warrants a higher level of privacy protection than unidentifiable information. Names, medical record numbers, and identifying photos are all considered identifiable information. Some information isn't considered identifiable by itself, but when combined with other information, can *become* identifiable. For example, a person's gender, address, or birth date alone aren't identifiable, but the situation changes when the three are combined.

It's also important to also consider the *sensitivity* of identifiable information. Identifiable health information is considered sensitive and warrants a higher level of protection. For instance, the harm caused by a data breach that exposes a patient's HIV status is considerably more severe than one that exposes their zip code. The level of protection should generally be proportionate to the sensitivity of the identifiable information.

Conversely, not all information that is collected about a patient is identifiable. For instance, most software routinely collects anonymous user information: device type, browser resolution, usage patterns, etc. This data is not identifiable data, so it's considered low risk and is subsequently not held to the same standard of privacy expectations as identifiable information.

Removing patient identifiers is a great way to transform information from high risk to low. Clinical researchers, for example, routinely remove individually identifiable information from datasets to protect patient privacy. If deidentified information can no longer be directly or indirectly linked back to an individual, then it's no longer identifiable and no longer warrants the same level of protection. In sum, the most important thing to remember is to protect identifiable health information more vigilantly than nonidentifiable nonhealth information.

Collecting and Sharing Information

If you determine that you need to store patient identifying information as part of your telehealth solution, you'll need to understand the limits to which information can be collected and shared. Privacy laws require practitioners to only collect and share the minimum necessary information to achieve the desired health benefit or to accomplish a specific purpose.[274]

Patients should know why their information is being collected, ideally at the time it's collected. Typically, this is done via blanket consent at the beginning of treatment. If you use blanket consent for telemedicine, make sure that it covers any telehealth-specific information not typically collected during in-person visits, especially if your sessions are recorded.

Though telemedicine has made it much easier for clinicians to record patient sessions, keeping a recording long term increases your risk of exposure. To reduce liability, many clinicians will delete the recording after it's served its purpose. The more patient information you have in different systems, the more you're obligated to manage, *and* the greater risk for hacking, ransomware, and more.

Sharing patient information with other providers, staff, and administrators is often necessary when providing healthcare. However, the information shared should be limited to only what's necessary, and only with those who need to know; a nurse treating a patient for a broken toe doesn't need access to a recent psychiatric evaluation. Likewise, the insurance company processing a payment for that broken toe doesn't need a patient's family history; the diagnosis and list of services rendered is all that's needed to pay the bill.

A description of how information will be used should be included in patient consent. While it's not possible to list everyone who may come in contact with the patient's information throughout the course of treatment, privacy regulations fortunately don't require this level of specificity as long those who access the data have a legitimate reason to do so.

Sharing patient information outside of healthcare settings without patient consent is almost always a bad idea. One of the more prominent recent examples of this involved Ashley Jacobs, the star of the reality show *Southern Charm*. While working as a home health-care aide in Charleston, South Carolina, Jacobs sent one of her fans a "thank you" video of herself while caring for a nonverbal pediatric patient. When the patient clearly appeared in the video, Jacobs was reported for a HIPAA violation, a situation that could have been avoided had she received permission from the patient's family.

Many should worry less about hackers than their clinical staff, because it's the staff that tend to be the greatest liability for unwanted information exposure. In 2008, after Britney Spears checked into a psychiatric unit at UCLA Medical Center, thirteen employees were fired and six physicians were suspended for snooping around in her medical records.[275] Another former employee faced up to ten years for leaking information about Farrah Fawcett's cancer diagnosis to the tabloids for $4,600. These cases apply to regular folks, too; even a nurse exploring the medical record of a neighbor without permission or a legitimate reason amounts to a HIPAA violation.

While it's generally a violation for a clinician, staff, or healthcare entity to share information without patient consent, remember that it's never a violation if patients choose to share *their own* health information. Some patients are more open with their health information on social media than others, and they're free to share what they like.

BUSINESS ASSOCIATES AGREEMENTS

When it comes to information flow, healthcare is deeply interconnected. Modern healthcare runs on a vast network of interconnected third parties to collect, manage, process, store, and present patient information. A clinician may use EHR software that uses a third-party data processor that itself runs on a third-party server. Patient information must flow effectively among these multiple services and subservices for the system to work.

Third-party services that manage patient data don't need additional patient consent as long as the information in question meets four criteria. First, it must fall under the purview of the original purpose and consent with the patient. Second, it must be limited to the extent necessary to accomplish its purposes. Third, it cannot be disclosed to unauthorized parties. Fourth, it must be protected to the same standard as the original clinician.

To codify this agreement, a business associates agreement (BAA) is signed between the patient's organization and connected services. Failure to have a BAA in place can result in hefty liabilities for failures. North Memorial Health Care of Minnesota was hit with a $1.55 million HIPAA violation fine after a laptop computer with unencrypted patient information was stolen from one of their associates. North Memorial didn't have a signed BAA with that associate, so they were on the hook for the full fine.

Understand that simply signing a BAA does not resolve your liability. Anybody can *say* they're HIPAA compliant before they sign a BAA, but healthcare clinicians need to make reasonable efforts to ensure that technologies, services, and subservices will *truly* keep their patient information safe. To do this, review your business associates' information privacy policies, ask for an independent HIPAA compliance assessment when in doubt, and most of all, avoid doing business with organizations that fail to demonstrate adequate compliance practices.

Sometimes HIPAA and a BAA aren't enough to keep patient information private from third-party services. Recently, a number of online DTC telemedicine services have come under increased scrutiny for passing identifying health information to third-party advertisers such as Google and Facebook for tracking purposes.[276] While the service claims that information entered on these intake forms is confidential and secure, some of the information passed to advertisers contains identifying information, including answers to health intake forms. Technically, this isn't a HIPAA violation. Since HIPAA governs interactions between clinicians and patients, information collected during a telehealth *company's* intake may not be protected by HIPAA, while the same information given to the *provider* would be. Clearly, HIPAA wasn't built for this situation, and the government continues to weigh its options.[277]

PATIENT ACCESS TO INFORMATION

If you do store patient information, you need to make that information accessible to them upon request; if it is not, you can be charged a fine. Patients have the right to request a copy of their data, to receive it in an intelligible format, and to get it within a reasonable timeframe. Denying patients copies of their health records, overcharging for copies, or failing to provide those records within thirty days is a violation of HIPAA. Cignet of Prince George's County found this out upon being fined $4.3 million for the forty-one separate occasions it refused to provide patients with copies of their own medical records.[278]

Remember that the more patient information you store across multiple systems, including telemedicine recordings, the more you have to release upon their request. In turn, the less patient information you store, the less you have to share with them.

Information privacy is of paramount importance in the modern world, and a constellation of laws and guidelines have been enacted to ensure information privacy. To be successful with telemedicine, do not store patient information unless you absolutely have to. If you do collect patient information, understand its nature and limit it to the minimum necessary. Sign a BAA with any telehealth technology you use and provide access to any patient information upon their request.

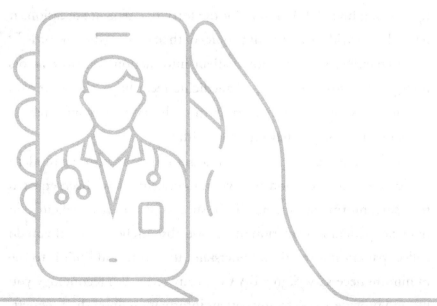

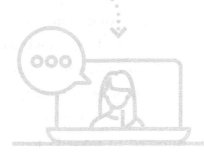

CHAPTER 20

Information Security

While you may be doing everything right to keep your patient information private, information won't stay private if it's not also secure. Recently, a hacking group known as The Dark Overlord engaged in a scheme that's becoming fairly common: exploiting unpatched security vulnerabilities among several healthcare organizations across the US to steal medical records and then offering them for ransom in exchange for Bitcoin.[279] If the healthcare organization refuses to pay, the hackers threaten to sell the data, leak it on the internet, and/or tip journalists about the breach to generate negative press. Organizations in turn will often pay hackers to protect the privacy of their patient information and hopefully avoid even larger fines, which further emboldens bad actors to pursue these kinds of schemes.

The extortion business has proven to be so successful that it's grown to include newer, more sophisticated tactics, many of which don't even require hackers to steal patient information. For instance, hackers will often breach networks, scan for vulnerabilities, and then attempt to extort money from the organization *before* disclosing the security flaws. It's manipulative and illegal, but it still happens.

Many hackers have even started using ransomware—a program that maliciously encrypts applications, computers, or databases—to block access until a ransom has been paid. This is exactly what happened to Ireland's public healthcare system, Health Service Executive (HSE), in May 2021: hackers used ransomware to block access to the national electronic health record system. Appointments had to be canceled en masse as the health system reverted temporarily back to paper records. Meanwhile, the hackers demanded a ransom of €16.5 million to decrypt the system.[280] The HSE chose not to pay the ransom and opted instead to restore their systems through backups. Within four months, 95 percent of servers and devices were back online, but the hackers still published confidential medical information for over five hundred patients. The total cost of the cyberattack and subsequent IT improvements exceeded €100 million.[281]

> **34 percent of healthcare organizations have allegedly been hit by ransomware attacks.**

Similarly, the University of Vermont Medical Center was hit by a ransomware program in 2020 that maliciously encrypted 1,300 servers and deposited malware on over 5,000 devices. To limit further damage, the information security team shut down all internet connections, including access to the EHR. For twenty-eight days, clinicians had to use paper records while they rebuilt the entire IT infrastructure from the ground up. It took several months and cost the Vermont hospital system $54 million, including lost revenue.[282]

They're far from alone: 34 percent of healthcare organizations have allegedly been hit by ransomware attacks.[283] In 2020 and 2021, at least

168 ransomware attacks affected a total of 1,763 clinics, hospitals, and healthcare organizations in the US.[282] It is such a common occurrence that the government now regularly publishes security notices on exceptionally aggressive ransomware groups targeting healthcare organizations.

In the end, *all* patient information must be secured, no matter where it is stored. If your telehealth solution is processing or storing patient information, you must guard it against unauthorized access, modification, or destruction. Given the rise in sophisticated attacks—to say nothing of curious employees—a strong security plan should include physical and technical safeguards and administrative controls to protect against unauthorized access.

Safeguards

At the most fundamental level, physical safeguards ensure that *physical* access to computers, servers, cables, routers, and other digital infrastructure is secure from unauthorized access. Physical controls, such as locking doors, Radio Frequency Identification (RFID) cards, and security cameras help to deter malicious or curious individuals from accessing things they shouldn't. Healthcare organizations using physical telemedicine carts or running their own video service in-house need to be particularly vigilant in ensuring their telemedicine equipment is physically secure at all times, even when not in use. Alternatively, software-based telemedicine solutions that use the cloud typically rely on servers located in secure data centers in which physical protections are already included with the service.

Likewise, there are other safeguards organizations use to protect against unauthorized *electronic* access to patient data. Whether the data is at rest or in transit, industry-standard encryption should be used to conceal patient information. Encryption is one of the most effective ways to prevent data breaches; even if accessed or stolen, encrypted information does not need to be reported if the decryption key was not stolen as well.

Malware and antivirus software should also be used to detect and block malicious code from capturing data via keyboard entry, microphone, or camera. Similarly, private networks with firewalls should be used, and network traffic should be actively monitored for signs of possible intrusions to stop exploits before they happen.

One of the most common security vulnerabilities is out-of-date software. Software companies generally do a good job of identifying and patching security vulnerabilities quickly, so it's important to conduct regular vulnerability scans and keep telehealth software and operating systems up to date. Finally, backing up system data is key to overcoming ransomware attacks because they can be used to restore a system after a clean and reset; just ensure that your backups are encrypted and regularly tested for data integrity.

AUTHENTICATION

Authentication is one of the most important aspects of technical security because it's where the most breaches occur. Most hackers don't need sophisticated software or skills to gain access to many systems; often, they can simply pretend to be someone they're not. A username and password is the only thing that stands between a hacker and patient information, so naturally, hackers spend a lot of effort trying to access passwords. The most common way hackers steal login credentials is through phishing emails, where hackers simply send an email with a link to a fake login screen for a familiar service. When you enter your username and password into the fake login screen, both go straight to the hacker, who then uses it to log in to your real account.

There are many other approaches to gaining access to passwords. Brute force attacks use trial and error to check a list of commonly used passwords until the correct one is found to login to your account. So if your password is something like "Password123," you should change it as soon as possible. Unfortunately, the widely used practice of eight character passwords with a combination of capital letters, numbers, and special characters is actually no longer recommended by the National Institute of Standards and Technology. The longer your password, the less susceptible it is to brute force attacks. With that in mind, "pumpkin-corvette-sprinkles" is significantly harder to hack than "Sprinkles123!"

Similarly, don't store passwords in an unencrypted text file on your desktop, which is precisely how The Dark Overlord gained access to the digital medical records at one clinic. Avoid writing your password on a sticky note and displaying it on your computer monitor, and don't share user accounts or passwords with others, especially digitally, as hackers could be monitoring your communication.

To combat unauthorized access due to a compromised password, two-factor authentication (2FA) provides an extra layer of protection. With 2FA enabled, logging into an account requires a password and an action (usually a temporary code) available only to you on a separate personal device, such as your phone. Biometric (fingerprint) and RFID cards are also both solid means of strengthening account authentication beyond passwords.

ADMINISTRATIVE SAFEGUARDS

Administrative safeguards are the final piece of the information security puzzle and should be documented, accessible, and reviewed regularly. Access to systems must be properly approved, monitored, and removed as appropriate. Employees need to be trained to ensure that safeguards are adhered to, and they should be aware of the latest security exploits and how to avoid falling victim to them.

Additionally, a logging system should be in place to monitor who's accessing what. Any telemedicine technology you use should have logging, either via workstations or within the software itself. At minimum, logs should identify the clinician and start/stop call times. Remember, if patient names are stored in the log file, then the log file itself contains patient health information and will need to be protected accordingly.

Organizations should also conduct regular security risk analyses and privacy impact assessments to root out vulnerabilities and to ensure that privacy and security protocols are being followed. One data breach involving 55,000 patients occurred when a laptop computer and unencrypted backup drive were stolen from the parked vehicle of an employee at the Cancer Care Group of Indiana. During the subsequent investigation, it became clear that the clinic never conducted a comprehensive risk assessment, which had allowed the risk to persist for years. Had they identified the risk after a proper assessment, protections could have been put into place to prevent the breach from occurring. In the end, they were fined $750,000 for the breach and the failure to perform a risk assessment.

Once security risks are identified, organizations must adhere to a vetted risk-management process to mitigate issues in a reasonable time frame. Knowing risks and failing to address them often yields stronger penalties; the University of Massachusetts Amherst was similarly fined $650,000 for failing to implement technical security measures for two years after an initial breach.

BE PRACTICAL

While all these security risks and mitigation strategies may feel daunting, you don't need to stress. Regulations such as HIPAA and GDPR are not overly prescriptive; they're deliberately vague to allow organizations to implement the safeguards in a reasonable and practical way. Also, the nature and amount of patient health information available should dictate the level of access controls used. Again, more sensitive patient information requires stronger safeguards.

The size of your organization, its technological capabilities, and your financial resources are all relevant considerations when crafting an information security plan. Small private practices with limited patient information aren't held to the same security standards as massive health systems with large amounts of highly sensitive patient health information. Likewise, a small primary care clinic isn't expected to have a dedicated security team, while large health systems with several hospitals should. It's worth noting that midsized organizations tend to incur the greatest risk; they're large enough to pay a healthy ransom but often small enough to lack a strong information security team. As a general rule, healthcare organizations should spend between 6 and14 percent of their annual IT budgets on security.

Before using a given telemedicine technology, verify it has appropriate information security safeguards in place by asking for third-party information security certifications—including SOC2, ISO27001, or FedRAMP—and by speaking to their privacy officer. Organizations shouldn't hide their privacy safeguards; it's always best to be transparent about patient data security practices and policies.

Accountability

Despite all the efforts to prevent a security breach, they can still happen. If there's any indication that unauthorized access, use, or disclosure of unprotected patient information has occurred, the first and most urgent step is to detect and stop the breach. If an employee accidentally shares the wrong patient file or a network analyst observes an anomaly in network traffic, they should immediately take action to stop further exposure and to limit the scale of the breach.

Every organization should have a privacy officer who is trained on how to properly investigate, mitigate, and respond to privacy breaches. Involve them as soon as possible to ensure that remediation is executed properly. An investigation generally will begin by interviewing involved parties, including those who committed the alleged violation, followed by any of those who received unintended information. If an electronic breach occurs, privacy officers will also gather evidence from system logs to determine the extent of exposure, the nature of information disclosed, and the source of the breach.

Their initial analysis will allow them to begin appropriate breach mitigation strategies, which can include terminating system access, changing passwords, remote-wiping devices, recovering disclosed information, or obtaining assurances from recipients that they will not use or abuse disclosed information. It may also entail making changes to information security policies, conducting additional employee training, issuing warnings, or imposing penalties on violators.

If a breach has indeed occurred—or at least is reasonably suspected—the organization must notify each patient affected. Different privacy laws have different notification requirements. To comply with HIPAA, each affected individual must be notified "without unreasonable delay," no later than sixty days after discovery.

Presence Health, one of the largest healthcare networks in Illinois, paid a $475,000 fine for notifying affected patients of a breach 101 days after it occurred, and their fine was increased after investigators discovered that patients hadn't been notified in a timely manner during other previous breaches.[284]

When a breach involves more than five hundred individuals, it must be reported to the media, who has a responsibility to report it to the public. Unsurprisingly, large-scale breach notifications can be costly. When the American Medical Collection Agency had to send seven million individuals breach notification letters, it cost them $3.8 million, on top of $400,000 for an outside IT firm to assist with their breach response.[285]

Notifying a patient of a breach is required only if the disclosure resulted in a privacy exposure. For example, if a hacker accesses a server only to find encrypted, inaccessible identifiable patient information, patients don't need to be notified. Similarly, medical records getting thrown in the trash without being shredded isn't a grave concern. Regardless, such breaches should still be reported to the privacy officer, who will ultimately determine whether a breach warrants further action.

> **Those who are entrusted to control and maintain patient information must be held accountable if a breach occurs.**

VIOLATION CONSEQUENCES

Those who are entrusted to control and maintain patient information must be held accountable if a breach occurs. While most breaches are handled and enforced internally, breaches exceeding five hundred patients also need to be reported to the Office of Civil Rights at Health and Human Services (HHS), who are tasked with enforcing

HIPAA regulations, also within sixty days.[y] HHS investigators will review the facts, will assess the impact, and may require corrective actions to mitigate future risks. They typically only investigate large-scale breaches because they don't have the resources to pursue minor infractions. At the time of writing, they're currently investigating some nine hundred privacy breaches from the last two years alone.[286]

As long as organizations are sincerely trying to protect information privacy, most HHS HIPAA investigations are resolved through voluntary corrective action or technical assistance. However, when a healthcare organization is found to be *purposefully* negligent, HHS can and will impose fines on a tiered system. The lowest fines are around $125 for violations in which the organization was unaware and could not have realistically been avoided. The largest fines amount to up to $60,000 in cases of "willful neglect," where no attempt was made to correct a known violation. HHS can even impose criminal penalties for HIPAA violations, including sentences of up to ten years in prison for stealing health information for personal gain or malicious intent.

In addition to HHS fines, healthcare organizations can also face civil lawsuits by affected patients. An orthopedic practice in Florida reached a $4 million settlement with their patients for failing to properly secure their information and notify them of a breach in a timely manner. In addition to being compensated for financial losses as a result of the breach, patients received three years of identity theft protection services, fraud assistance, and identity restoration services.[287]

Perhaps the greatest damage to an organization after an information breach comes down to reputation and the subsequent loss of business. One study found that the share value of publicly traded

---

y   If a breach affects fewer than five hundred individuals, the covered entity may notify OCR on an annual basis.

companies dropped following the disclosure of a data breach.[288] When one medical debt company lost three of its largest clients after a breach, the company had to file for bankruptcy.[285]

In the end, information won't stay private if it isn't secured, so you must guard your telehealth solution against unauthorized access. To be successful with telemedicine, ensure appropriate physical and technical safeguards are in place to keep your patients' information secure, use strong passwords and authentication processes, ensure that safeguards are properly documented and followed, and be accountable when a security breach happens.

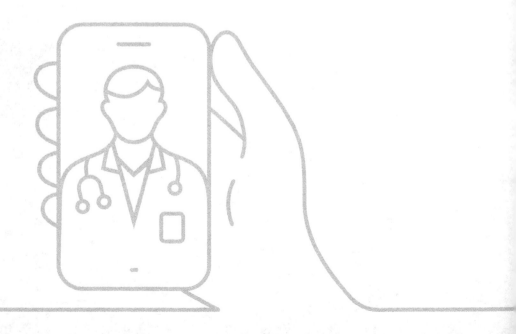

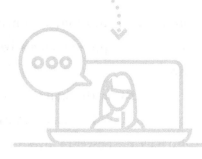

CHAPTER 21

Medical Boards

W hile the preceding chapters in this section have largely focused on compliance regarding laws established by elected legislative bodies, this one will focus more on regulations, policies, and recommendations created by professional and organizational bodies (e.g., medical boards). You'll notice differences in the power of these regulations compared to the law and the ability of clinicians to influence them in favor of telehealth when necessary. States and medical boards have a lot of power and influence over telemedicine rules and regulations, so to be successful, it's important to understand the limits and constraints of their power.

Medical boards were originally created in the nineteenth century to protect the public from rampant medical quackery. States first granted incipient medical boards the power to create policies, rules, and standards to govern the profession for the general safety and protection of the public. To this day, the right to practice medicine is a privilege granted by state medical boards through a license. With a license, a clinician has authority to diagnose and treat patients, prescribe medication, administer treatment, perform surgical procedures, and present themselves as officially authorized to practice medicine.

Boards set the standards and requirements and then verify that the doctors in their states continue to meet those standards. Boards also have the power to investigate complaints and enforce their regulations with penalties such as reprimand, probation, fines, suspension, and revocation of licenses. Ultimately, clinicians take an oath to do no harm, and medical boards have the authority to ensure that happens.

In some cases, enforcement can lead to criminal action and incarceration, even for out-of-state clinicians. When Stanford freshman John McKay unexpectedly committed suicide by exhaust in his mother's garage, the autopsy found alcohol and fluoxetine in his system. Further investigation showed that he had obtained the over-the-counter antidepressant through an online pharmacy, where he'd simply filled out an online questionnaire and received the drug in the mail. John's online prescription request was sent to psychiatrist Christian Hagesth, MD, a subcontractor, who resided in and was only licensed to practice medicine in Colorado. Dr. Hagesth had never met John, nor had he established a clinician-patient relationship; he simply reviewed John's questionnaire and signed the order.[289]

While doing so didn't violate any laws at the time in and of itself, many states were seeking a way to clamp down on harmful unregulated "pill mills" that were flourishing on the web.[z] California couldn't go after the online pharmacy for their role in McKay's death. However, since Dr. Hagesth wasn't licensed to practice medicine in California, he was charged with a felony offense for practicing medicine in California without a license.

---

z   See chapter 17.

Dr. Hagesth and his attorney claimed that because he wasn't in the state when the crime was committed, the law didn't apply. The California courts didn't accept that argument, and Dr. Hagesth was ultimately found guilty. The sixty-eight-year-old, semiretired doctor was sentenced to nine months in prison, given a $4,000 fine, and gave up his Colorado medical license. The case has served as a warning to anyone providing care to a patient in another state ever since.

Teladoc versus the Texas Medical Board

The legal battle between Teladoc and the Texas Medical Board was one of the most pivotal sagas in telemedicine history. In 2010, the medical board made an amendment to their regulations requiring Texas physicians to conduct in-person physical examinations in order to establish a proper provider-patient relationship.[290] The move effectively eliminated Teladoc's ability to deliver their service, which was provided primarily by telephone at the time.

For several months, the Dallas-based Teladoc tried to work with the Texas Medical Board, but to little avail. Teladoc ultimately saw no other course of action but to take the matter to court. The State Court of Texas ultimately saw the board's behavior as unnecessarily restrictive, ruled in Teladoc's favor, and issued a temporary restraining order preventing enforcement of the medical board's rule. The Texas Medical Board swiftly appealed the decision, but after a four-year-long appeals process, the appeals court upheld the original decision.

Despite the court's ruling, the medical board promptly issued a punitive "emergency" rule defining "acceptable medical practice" as an in-person physical examination and declaring provider-patient relationships formed online or by phone as inadequate. Again, Teladoc obtained a temporary injunction against the rule in state court.

Undaunted, the board went through its own formal rulemaking process to create the Texas Medical Practices Act, which required face-to-face visits for physicians to write prescriptions for patients, regardless of medical necessity. Two weeks later, Teladoc filed suit in response, asserting that the medical board was violating antitrust law as well as the commerce clause of the US Constitution. The board attempted to get the suit dismissed, claiming immunity from antitrust liability as a quasi-state entity.

At this point, precedent became relevant. Two years earlier, the US Supreme Court had dealt with a similar case involving teeth-whitening services in North Carolina. The State Board of Dental Examiners had sent threatening letters to nondentists who were offering teeth whitening services, claiming that they were illegally engaging in the practice of dentistry and thus violating the North Carolina Dental Practice Act.[291] After hearing the case, the US Supreme Court ultimately ruled that while the dental board was a state agency, it was operated by market participants and elected by other market participants, and thus functioned as a private actor that did not qualify for state-action immunity. In other words, as a professional organization composed of competing dental clinicians, the organization was capable of conspiring with itself.

> **The law declared that the standard of care provided by telemedicine was the same as if it was delivered in person.**

That Supreme Court ruling paved the way for Texas courts to side with Teladoc. Back in Texas, the Federal Trade Commission sent a letter to the court criticizing the Texas Medical Board for misinterpreting case law and then united with the Department of Justice in support of Teladoc.[292] The Texas Medical Board dropped its motion to dismiss the suit but vowed to continue to fight the suit and for their right to regulate their industry as they saw fit.

To put the matter to rest, in May of 2017, the Texas State Legislature unanimously passed a telemedicine law making it legal in the state of Texas to establish a doctor-patient relationship solely via telemedicine, *without* the need for an in-person exam.[293] The law declared that the standard of care provided by telemedicine was the same as if it was delivered in person. It prohibited medical boards from imposing a more restrictive standard of care for telemedicine services and prohibited health plans from excluding coverage for telemedicine services solely because they weren't preceded by a face-to-face consultation. This outcome set a precedent in favor of telemedicine that's still relevant today. Teladoc dropped its suit, and telehealth has flourished in Texas ever since.

State Laws in the Modern Age

Many medical board policies and regulations were created in the first half of the twentieth century, before interstate travel and communication were widespread. As a result, many don't exactly jibe with the way modern healthcare is practiced today, especially when it comes to telehealth. The issues particularly compound in terms of patient and provider location.

For instance, a clinician is allowed to meet with a patient from another state at their clinic if the patient crossed a state line to get there. However, when that same patient returns home, that clinician cannot provide care to them by telemedicine, or even deliver a home visit, unless they're licensed to practice in that patient's state. When the state of Virginia rolled back Covid licensing exemptions, Johns

Hopkins Medicine in Maryland had to quickly notify more than a thousand of their Virginia patients that their telehealth appointments were "no longer feasible" because their treating clinicians were not licensed to practice in Virginia.[294]

There's also a difference between the *residence* and *presence* of the patient to consider. If a given patient is temporarily on vacation in another state, forgets their medication or falls ill, and wants to consult with their clinician back home, it's the clinician's professional and ethical duty to first protect the patient from harm by helping them or referring them to a local hospital. Technically, the clinician must be licensed in whatever state the patient is in to provide care legally, but it's unlikely that the state board will know or care; they have more important things to worry about. In fact, Iowa, Kansas, Connecticut, and Oregon have laws explicitly allowing care to be provided by out-of-state clinicians to their established patients who are in their state temporarily.

> **Once you've seen one medical board, you've seen one medical board.**

But when an established patient permanently moves to another state and establishes residency there, clinicians then need to seriously determine whether it makes sense to get licensed in that state or help the patient transition to a new, local clinician.

Once you've seen one medical board, you've seen one medical board; they're all as unique as the states they represent, with their own personalities, interests, and priorities. Every state has different rules, and they change constantly. Nothing highlights the inconsistency across states better than what happened in response to Covid. When qualified healthcare clinicians were needed most to respond to the health emergency, many medical board regulations became a barrier to care.

Fortunately, all fifty states issued orders allowing out-of-state clinicians to perform telehealth visits with their residents. But that's about where the unanimity ended. Fifty states solved the same problem in fifty different ways.[295] Many states, like South Carolina, simply waived license requirements. Others, like Ohio and Rhode Island, kept original laws in place but suspended enforcement. Most states allowed licensed clinicians from other states to practice in their states. New York and Wisconsin even allowed licensed Canadian clinicians to practice in their states. Hawaii allowed clinicians who were previously licensed but no longer current or active clinicians to engage in telehealth. Alabama created temporary special-purpose licenses for telemedicine. Arkansas and Pennsylvania gave temporary licenses to clinicians from adjoining states. It goes on and on.

As Covid receded, more changes followed. New Mexico and Arizona made their Covid license exemptions permanent and allowed licensed clinicians from other states to legally practice within their borders going forward. Delaware made an exception for out-of-state mental healthcare clinicians, who are still allowed to treat patients in their state. Virginia rescinded and then reinstituted telehealth waivers. Tennessee is perhaps the most confusing of all; its osteopathic board continues to issue telemedicine licenses, while the state medical board *eliminated* telemedicine licensure.

Medical boards have great authority to adapt the law to changes in environment, emergencies, and more, so don't be afraid to petition them for changes when they make sense. They're *intended* to be malleable, especially when you can show when their rules harm patients. Additionally, the Emergency Management Assistance Compact (EMAC) agreement, of which all states and territories are members, was created to enable state-to-state assistance during governor-declared states of emergency. It states that responders and clinicians using their professional skills at the request of another state "shall be deemed licensed, certified, or permitted by the state request-ing assistance to render aid involving such skill to meet a declared emergency or disaster." Relatedly, licensed professionals who are "fed-eralized" during a disaster as members of disaster medical assistance teams or via the US Public Health Service also do not require state licensure.[296]

The federal government can supersede state medical boards in certain situations. For instance, in December 2020, the 2005 Public Readiness and Emergency Preparedness (PREP) Act was amended by Congress to prevent state and local governments from enforcing regulations that keep qualified health professionals from delivering specific Covid-related services, including by telemedicine. Healthcare clinicians providing Covid care can do so with the protection of the federal government.

Additionally, clinicians providing care via telehealth on behalf of the federal government have their own rules. The Department of Veterans Affairs allows clinicians to practice within the scope and requirements of VA employment "regardless of state requirements that interfere with their practice." Similarly, clinicians for the Department of Defense and Indian Health Services only need a single state license to practice in any state on behalf of the federal government. Care delivered at federal prisons works in a similar way, though in-state prisons and county jails, clinicians must be licensed in the state where the patient is located and receiving care.

Finally, clinician-clinician consultation, in which a clinician seeks advice and expertise from another clinician regarding their patient, is another interesting licensing case. Consulted clinicians do not need to be licensed in the state where the patient resides as long as two things are true. First, the in-state consulting clinician must be responsible for clinician-patient relationship and must hold ultimate decision-making authority. Second, the out-of-state consulted clinician must be licensed in their own state. This is how peer consultation companies like AristaMD and RubiconMD, which provide broad online access to specialists for primary care clinicians, are able to provide their services nationwide without requiring their clinicians to be licensed everywhere. This is also how services like tele-stroke work, allowing specialized tertiary medical systems to connect to smaller rural hospitals, even ones outside their state.

Getting Licensed

Most clinicians traditionally are only licensed to practice in one state—the one where they and their patients reside. This works fine for most clinicians. The decision to get an additional license is often born out of practicality and necessity, such as clinicians who live near state borders or who have moved and opened practices in new states. Most clinicians need only one or two licenses. In most cases, the process to obtain them is fairly easy and straightforward: when you need a new license, you fill out an application, demonstrate that you meet their requirements, pay an application fee, and then get the license. Most license application requirements are the same, regardless of state.

However, if you're a clinician who wants to practice across multiple states or the entire country using telehealth, this process quickly becomes burdensome. Getting all boards from coast to coast to agree has been like herding cats, but fortunately, many boards recognized the problem[297] and have created the Interstate Medical Licensure Compact with the Federation of State Medical Boards in an attempt to streamline the licensing process. To get multiple licenses, physicians simply complete one application and pay the fee for each state.

In 2017, eighteen states joined immediately. The number has doubled since, and every state will likely become a member with time. However, as of 2021, only 0.6 percent of physicians have used the compact to obtain a license in another state, presumably due to lack of necessity during Covid. Getting multiple licenses is also costly; in addition to paying to be part of the compact ($700), each state requires clinicians to pay a licensing fee and renew every two years.

Several other healthcare professional licensing compacts use the principle of reciprocity, which is similar to how driver's licenses work. When you have a driver's license from one state, you're legally able to operate a motor vehicle in all states, obeying the laws of each state, but without needing a separate driver's license for each. The Nurse Licensure Compact allows nurses residing and licensed in a member state to receive a single multistate license which is valid in thirty-seven other states. The Psychology Interjurisdictional Compact likewise allows psychologists in participating jurisdictions to practice across state lines, and the Counseling Compact will permit the same for professional counselors. These compacts greatly expand the availability of qualified health professionals to the benefit of patients, and we hope to see more of them for those practicing medicine.[298] Given the shortage of qualified professionals in many parts of the country, states would be wise to increase access to qualified healthcare professionals within their borders.

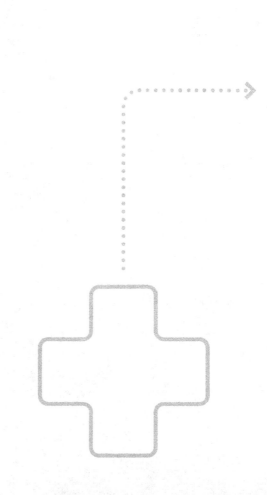

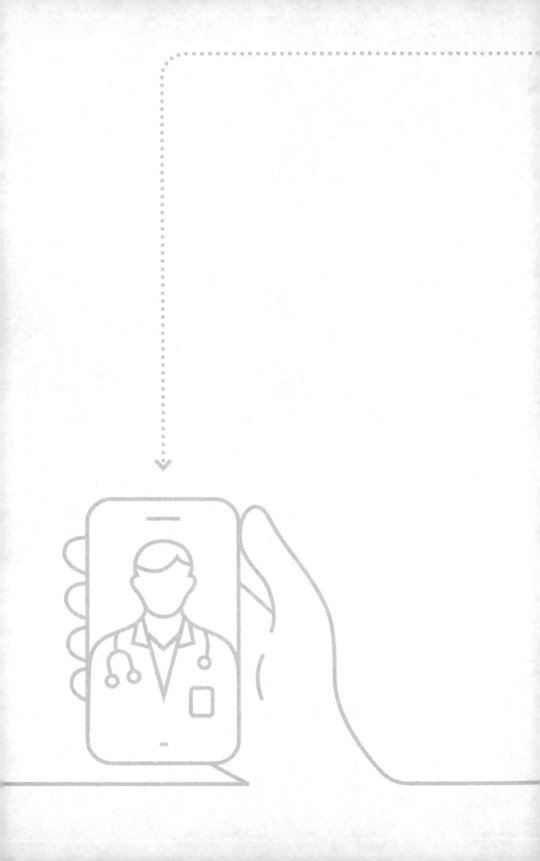

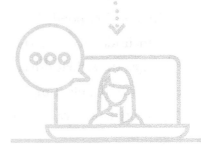

CHAPTER 22

Organizational Compliance

n early 2013, while I was a PhD student in biomedical informatics at the University of Utah, I created an early version of Doxy.me to use in a remote prenatal care clinical research study. I had to get the blessing of the director of telehealth for permission to use my app for the study. While giving him a demo, he smugly replied that it wasn't HIPAA compliant and therefore couldn't be used.

Surprised by his response, I asked "Why?"

"Because telemedicine apps need the patients to have a username and password," he responded.

I was familiar with security requirements and doubted his response, so again I asked, "Why?"

Like a wise father speaking to his son, he then told me, "You need to verify that the patient on the call is really that patient, and to do that, they have to create an account and set up a password.

To this, I responded with a leading question: "How do patients verify their identity for in-person appointments?"

"They show their driver's license to the receptionist."

On cue, I pulled my driver's license from my wallet and held it up to my laptop camera so it could be clearly seen on his screen. "Like this?"

At this, he was suddenly dumbfounded. Up to that point, nobody had ever challenged him on his assumption. Every other telemedicine technology used at the University of Utah at that time required patients to create usernames and passwords. "I'll have to get back to you," he said.

I eventually discovered that the Center for Telehealth had inherited the university's digital software applications policy for patient authentication. Granted, requiring a patient to enter a username and password is a legitimate way to verify identity in digital health apps, but in cases where there's a real-time video interaction with a patient, the requirement is unnecessary; a clinician can verify they're indeed seeing the correct patient simply by seeing and interacting with them as they would in person. Within a month, the requirement was rescinded for real-time video, and Doxy.me was being used by obstetricians to virtually meet with pregnant moms for prenatal care, with the added protocol that a doctor must confirm the patient's identity by driver's license at the start of every call.

> **Some rules and policies set by organizations are dumb, especially if they predate new technology and are adopted thoughtlessly.**

That experience taught me a few things. First, some rules and policies set by organizations are dumb, especially if they predate new technology and are adopted thoughtlessly. We've all faced obscure organizational policies that just don't make sense. All organizations have policies, ranging from employee conduct to information security, and in reality, most of us have never seen or even know about them. Most healthcare organizational policies are created to achieve accreditation and certifications, such as the joint commission for patient quality, or SOC2 for information security. The truth about most of these policies is that they're typically just carbon copies of some other organization's policies and procedures.

While these accreditation and certification have standards that must be followed, specifically *how* they're followed is usually left up to the organization. Often, organizations default to taking a stricter approach than required. Many find it easier to adopt a blanket approach, being overly restrictive to avoid all possible risk, to the detriment of usability.

The second thing I learned is that, *unlike* laws, organizational policies can be malleable, especially if you talk to the right people. I've found that organizational policies tend to be the strictest in terms of requirements *and* most malleable when changes are needed. If a policy's enforcement hinders your ability to provide telemedicine effectively, you can often work with the person enforcing the policy to understand it and the standard it's trying to uphold. By referring back to the original standard, whether it's for HIPAA or an accreditation standard, you can understand its real intent and ideally come up with alternative ways to uphold it without interfering with your ability to practice telemedicine. You may have to seek higher authority from senior leadership to gain an exception to a policy, but if you go in with sound justification and a reasonable alternative plan to meet the standard, you're more likely to be successful.

Sadly, working with enforcers doesn't always work out. For several years, an information security analyst at MUSC restricted the use of Doxy.me to "research purposes only" because a dated organizational security policy required telemedicine solutions to be hosted on MUSC's own on-site servers. Despite this not being a HIPAA requirement, and the fact that most of the health IT was already on the cloud, we couldn't get the analyst to budge. Eventually, the arbitrary requirement was rescinded when Covid hit and the existing infrastructure wasn't able to handle the dramatic spike in call volume. They've been using Doxy.me for clinical purposes without issue ever since.

Informed Consent

Informed consent is the legal and ethical process by which patients are informed of the treatment, procedure, and intervention they receive. Patients have every right to receive information, ask questions, and understand the relevant facts in the name of making well-informed decisions. They should be made thoroughly aware of expected benefits *and* possible risks, available alternatives and their implications, the proposed course of action, and how their data will be used.

While there's broad consensus for the necessity of medical consent, different state laws, accreditation organizations, ethicists, and lawyers all have different ideas regarding when and how consent should be done, and for what purposes. As a result, there's considerable variability in how consent is handled between organizations. Most consent in healthcare is implied or verbal, but signed consent at the start of a clinician-patient relationship is generally a good idea. It's even more essential in cases that involve a high-risk or adverse outcome, invasive surgical procedures, high-risk medications, or experimental studies.

Conversely, informed consent in research has a higher bar because research studies are experimental in nature. To protect patients from harm and to protect organizations from liability, patients need to be fully informed of potential risks for any treatment that falls outside of standard of care. Back when telemedicine was new, healthcare organizations and even some states required written consent that explained what telehealth is and its potential risks. As telemedicine adoption has expanded, many organizations have updated their consent forms to include telemedicine as an option that doesn't require separate consent. In the end, it's best to check state laws to understand if explicit consent for telemedicine is still required in your state.

Generally, consent should be granted before a patient receives care, but obtaining it in writing can be challenging via telemedicine. There are many ways to obtain written consent digitally, including patient portals, document-signing services like DocuSign, and mailing or emailing consent forms. Each approach has its own strengths and weaknesses.

When I first arrived at MUSC in 2014, clinical researchers were struggling to obtain consent from participants statewide for telemedicine studies. The MUSC Institutional Review Board (IRB) required obtaining research consent in person, despite the fact that the study's research interventions were being done entirely remotely by video. Furthermore, the IRB wanted researchers to review the consent document with participants to ensure they understood every paragraph and refused to allow asynchronous consent because they wanted participants to have real-time interactions during the entire process. They were also hypersensitive to any possible errors on the consent forms, including typos or missing dates, as these would invalidate the document and require the researcher to start it over from scratch.

An initial attempt was made to email consent documents to participants with a corresponding review phone call, but that soon turned into a logistical nightmare because participants had to print documents (while most didn't have computers or printers), schedule a phone call, ensure their signatures were in the right places, and then scan or mail the forms back in a timely manner. Every stage was prone to failure, and on top of that, the IRB was concerned about verifying the IDs of signees.

As a result, research participants and staff ended up having to drive several hours just to complete a consent document. Furthermore, every time the consent needed to be updated, which happened frequently, the whole process had to start over from scratch. The regulations of the IRB made it extremely burdensome for researchers to recruit participants, particularly in the rural areas that the related grants were specifically trying to address.

After understanding everyone's needs, we proposed creating a way for researchers to obtain consent from participants in real time using telemedicine, which we called "teleconsent."[299] Using the Doxy.me platform, teleconsent allows researchers to verify participants by video, then walk through consent documents together. When it came time to sign the document, participants

> **Teleconsent ultimately combined the convenience of telemedicine with the IRB's strict requirements.**

could either sign with their mouse or use a "photo signature," which took a picture of the participant from their video feed combined with their name, date, and IP address. This created a legally verifiable signature that complied with the requirements of Title 21 CFR Part 11 subpart C.

Teleconsent ultimately combined the convenience of telemedicine with the IRB's strict requirements and has gone on to receive several grants from the NIH to further its development. Teleconsent is increasingly being used by researchers and healthcare organizations in the clinical setting as well. While the full capabilities of teleconsent are not necessary every time consent is required, in cases where a higher bar is required, it's a convenient option to have.

Every organization has its own rules, and while rules at the organizational level tend to be the most strict, they're also often the most malleable. To be successful with telemedicine, understand the purposes for which organizational policies are made and propose reasonable alternatives when any inhibit your ability to practice telemedicine.

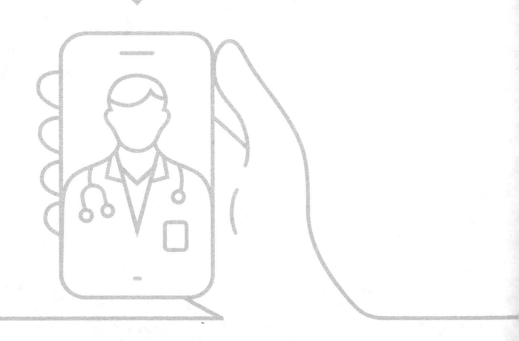

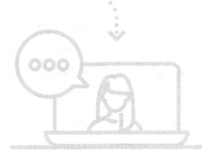

CONCLUSION

Telehealth has the potential to revolutionize healthcare delivery and will undoubtedly play an increasingly important role in the health and well-being of patients around the world. However, this won't happen unless *everyone* is successful: patients, clinicians, administrators, organizations, payers, and governments alike. We don't want you to just use telemedicine; we want you to be successful with it. The goal of this book is to help you go from simply using telemedicine to *thriving* through your use of it.

For patients to be successful with telemedicine, it needs to be used to overcome the many systemic, geographic, and social barriers that limit access to healthcare. Patients need to receive care by telemedicine in a safe, effective, and patient-centric way, and their care must be the same or better as they currently receive it in person. Finally, patients themselves need to be satisfied with telehealth and receive it in a way they prefer.

For clinicians to be successful, telehealth must help them deliver high quality care more effectively, increase their satisfaction, and reduce burnout. Clinicians also need to conduct remote exams with patients in an effective and professional manner. Clinician success is highly tied to organizational success, which requires alignment to what patients and clinicians need. Effective implementation from start to finish, including training and evaluation, will be necessary for a telemedicine program to be successful.

To successfully use telehealth technology, the right technology needs to be used for the right use case, and it must integrate seamlessly with current workflows. Every technology component must work together to achieve high call quality. There are many ways in which technology can fail, and how they're handled is key.

Telemedicine must also be financially viable to be successful. Understanding what motivates government, insurance, employers, and sometimes patients is key to getting paid for providing telemedicine. On the other side of the equation, telemedicine can and should also be used to cut the cost of providing healthcare.

Finally, to stay out of trouble as telehealth evolves, it's important to comply with laws and regulations. Clinicians need to avoid activities that can hinder their success, like malpractice and fraud. Understanding prescription laws and following privacy and security laws will help protect you *and* your patients. Learning to work with medical boards and their regulations will minimize avoidable issues, as will keeping up with ever-changing state regulations.

By following the strategies outlined in this book, healthcare organizations can successfully implement telehealth and realize its full potential, but this book alone may not be enough to make you successful. You will also need to stay up to date. To this end, we've created a free online resource, www.TelehealthSuccess.com, where we'll publish articles, podcasts, videos, blog posts, research publications, success manuals for specific specialties, updated information on reimbursement, regulatory guides, and material related to training and best practices. We also recognize that some of the advice we've provided may be harder to implement than what the book alone can provide. If and when you need the assistance of experts, we've also provided a list of vetted telehealth experts whose services we wholeheartedly recommend.

A book on how to be successful with telemedicine can never be fully complete; we'll always be learning, and the field is always changing. Healthcare relies heavily on reviewing, analyzing, and translating evidence from research into practice. We're actively involved in telehealth research and want to learn from you. As you begin implementing these principles, we want to know what worked and what didn't. We want to know the changes you made to help your particular practice thrive. We invite you to share with others to help them overcome the same challenges you may

> **We'll always be learning, and the field is always changing.**

have faced, if only to find the right answer faster and to avoid repeated failures. Everyone benefits by learning together. As we learn how to be successful together, we can all help advance the field of telemedicine faster and collectively avoid mistakes.

Additionally, policy and decision makers, payers, and any and all others who create laws, policy, and regulations rely on data to make informed decisions that benefit telemedicine. Research and data are critical to convince these individuals of the value of telemedicine so that they can go on to create policies that benefit the industry as a whole.

Sound research principles and techniques are necessary to ensure valid results. Not everyone has the luxury of in-house researchers to help put the information together in a reliable and convincing format. We can connect you with PhD-level researchers who focus exclusively on telemedicine research and can help you publish your research, write grants, and generally get your findings out in the world to help *others* be successful with telemedicine.

As you gain experience and become more successful with telehealth, we invite you to also share your successes with your colleagues. Professional organizations play a critical role in establishing standards, training, and guidelines within a specialty. With broader adoption of telehealth, many specialty organizations are looking at how telehealth is used within their specialty and how to plan for its use in the future. They wisely look to their members to set the standard for telehealth clinical care and beyond.

For instance, the American College of Emergency Physicians was instrumental in allowing clinician voices in advocating for better reimbursement during the pandemic, as well as defining a specific role for telehealth as part of emergency measures. ER physicians have also worked on defining what tele-emergency medicine will look like, who will comprise staff, what skills are and will be needed, what research is most pressing, and how to fill the many gaps in the field. Involvement in these organizations can be instrumental in expanding the principles of telehealth success within your field. We invite you to be an active participant and advocate for telehealth success among your colleagues and at professional organizations.

Finally, many laws, policies, and regulations will contribute to the growth of telehealth. It is important for the future of telehealth that those who are successful with it speak up for and advocate for its continued support *and* advocate for nonrestrictive policies. It will take all of us to contact policy makers, legislators, payers, and administrators and leaders of individual organizations to ensure that telehealth remains successful.

In the future, when we look back at this time, we'll likely see this moment as the moment telehealth started to fundamentally transform healthcare. The healthcare of the future stands to be more accessible, more convenient, more affordable, and more equitable. What an amazing movement to be a part of! Yet the future that we all envision and desire won't come to pass if we don't embrace the principles required to be successful *and* share that knowledge with others. While it starts at the individual level, collectively, we can shape the future of healthcare.

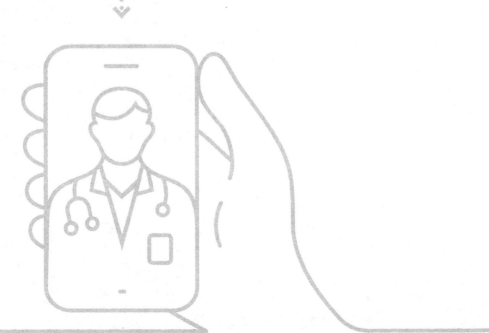

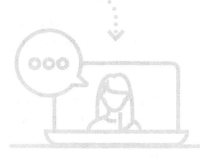

REFERENCES

1. Bestsennyy, O., Gilbert, G., Harris, A. & Rost, J. Telehealth: a quarter-trillion-dollar post-COVID-19 reality? https://www.mckinsey.com/industries/healthcare/our-insights/telehealth-a-quarter-trillion-dollar-post-covid-19-reality (2020).

2. Anderson, B. Doctor infected with COVID-19 continues to treat patients virtually. FOX 29 News Philadelphia. https://www.fox29.com/news/doctor-infected-with-covid-19-continues-to-treat-patients-virtually (2020).

3. Lee, F., Maggiore, P. & Chung, K. Self-management of an inferior ST-segment elevation myocardial infarction. *N. Engl. J. Med.* **378**, 960–962 (2018).

4. Goldschmidt, G. & Pate, M. A. Every year nearly 6 million people die in developing countries from low quality healthcare—this is how we help them. World Economic Forum. https://www.weforum.org/agenda/2019/11/effects-and-costs-of-poor-quality-healthcare/ (2019).

5.   Ngo, T. A survey of patient satisfaction with telemedicine during the COVID-19 pandemic at a student-run free clinic. *Free Clinic Research Collective* **6** (2020).

6.   American Hospital Association. *Rural Report.* https://www.aha.org/system/files/2019-02/rural-report-2019.pdf (2019).

7.   Dickman, S. L. *et al.* Trends in health care use among Black and White persons in the US, 1963–2019. *JAMA Netw Open* **5**, e2217383 (2022).

8.   Al Kasab, S., Adams, R. J., Debenham, E., Jones, D. J. & Holmstedt, C. A. Medical University of South Carolina. Telestroke: a telemedicine facilitated network for stroke treatment in South Carolina—a progress report. *Telemed. J. E. Health.* **23**, 674–677 (2017).

9.   Simpson, A. N. *et al.* Population health indicators associated with a statewide telestroke program. *Telemed. J. E. Health.* **26**, 1126–1133 (2020).

10. Butzner, M. & Cuffee, Y. Telehealth interventions and outcomes across rural communities in the United States: narrative review. *J. Med. Internet Res.* **23**, e29575 (2021).

11. Arora, S. *et al.* Outcomes of treatment for hepatitis C virus infection by primary care providers. *N. Engl. J. Med.* **364**, 2199–2207 (2011).

12. Osei-Twum, J.-A. *et al.* Impact of Project ECHO on patient and community health outcomes: a scoping review. *Acad. Med.* **97**, 1393–1402 (2022).

13. Zong, J., Zong, J. B. J. & Batalova, J. The limited English proficient population in the United States in 2013. Migrationpolicy.org. https://www.migrationpolicy.org/article/limited-english-proficient-population-united-states-2013 (2015).

14. Joshi, C. *et al.* A narrative synthesis of the impact of primary health care delivery models for refugees in resettlement countries on access, quality and coordination. *Int. J. Equity Health* **12**, 88 (2013).

15. Marshall, E. G., Wong, S. T., Haggerty, J. L. & Levesque, J.-F. Perceptions of unmet healthcare needs: what do Punjabi and Chinese-speaking immigrants think? A qualitative study. *BMC Health Serv. Res.* **10**, 46 (2010).

16. Chandrashekar, P., Zhang, R., Leung, M. & Jain, S. H. Impact of patient-physician language concordance on healthcare utilization. *J. Gen. Intern. Med.* **37**, 2120–2122 (2022).

17. Basu, G., Costa, V. P. & Jain, P. Clinicians' obligations to use qualified medical interpreters when caring for patients with limited English proficiency. *AMA Journal of Ethics* **19**, 245–252 (2017).

18. Al Shamsi, H., Almutairi, A. G., Al Mashrafi, S. & Al Kalbani, T. Implications of language barriers for healthcare: a systematic review. *Oman Med. J.* **35**, e122 (2020).

19. Doxy. Me Inc. Doxy.me extends telemedicine's reach to 88% of the world's population. *PR Newswire.* https://www.prnewswire.com/news-releases/doxyme-extends-telemedicines-reach-to-88-of-the-worlds-population-301636792.html (2022).

20. Mussallem, A. *et al.* Making virtual health care accessible to the deaf community: findings from the telehealth survey. *J. Telemed. Telecare* 1357633X221074863 (2022).

21. United Nations, D. of E. & Social Affairs, P. D. Population Division. *World Population Ageing 2019: Highlights* (ST/ESA/SER. A/430). (2019).

22. Doraiswamy, S., Jithesh, A., Mamtani, R., Abraham, A. & Cheema, S. Telehealth use in geriatrics care during the COVID-19 pandemic—

A scoping review and evidence synthesis. *Int. J. Environ. Res. Public Health* **18**, (2021).

23. Voice of the Consumer *et al.* Consumer adoption of telemedicine in 2021. Rock Health. https://rockhealth.com/insights/consumer-adoption-of-telemedicine-in-2021/ (2021).

24. Bhatia, R. *et al.* Older adults' perspectives on primary care telemedicine during the COVID-19 pandemic. *J. Am. Geriatr. Soc.* **70**, 3480–3492 (2022).

25. Jacqueline, L. & Maria, V. *Telemedicine Use among Adults: United States, 2021.* https://stacks.cdc.gov/view/cdc/121435 (2022) doi:10.15620/cdc:121435.

26. Xiong, J. & Muraki, S. Thumb performance of elderly users on smartphone touchscreen. *Springerplus* **5**, 1218 (2016).

27. Mao, A. *et al.* Barriers to telemedicine video visits for older adults in independent living facilities: mixed methods cross-sectional needs assessment. *JMIR Aging* **5**, e34326 (2022).

28. Annaswamy, T. M., Verduzco-Gutierrez, M. & Frieden, L. Telemedicine barriers and challenges for persons with disabilities: COVID-19 and beyond. *Disabil. Health J.* **13**, 100973 (2020).

29. Williams, D. R. & Rucker, T. D. Understanding and addressing racial disparities in health care. *Health Care Financ. Rev.* **21**, 75–90 (2000).

30. Anastos-Wallen, R. E. *et al.* Primary care appointment completion rates and telemedicine utilization among Black and Non-Black patients from 2019 to 2020. *Telemed. J. E. Health.* **28**, 1786–1795 (2022).

31. Scheer, J. *et al.* Racial and ethnic differences in outcomes of a 12-week digital rehabilitation program for musculoskeletal pain: prospective longitudinal cohort study. *J. Med. Internet Res.* **24**, e41306 (2022).

32. Snyder, J. E. *et al.* Black representation in the primary care physician workforce and its association with population life expectancy and mortality rates in the US. *JAMA Netw Open* **6**, e236687 (2023).

33. Pinquart, M. & Sörensen, S. Differences between caregivers and non-caregivers in psychological health and physical health: a meta-analysis. *Psychol. Aging* **18**, 250–267 (2003).

34. Eberly, L. A. *et al.* Patient characteristics associated with telemedicine access for primary and specialty ambulatory care during the COVID-19 pandemic. *JAMA Netw Open* **3**, e2031640 (2020).

35. Reed, M. E. *et al.* Patient characteristics associated with choosing a telemedicine visit vs office visit with the same primary care clinicians. *JAMA Netw Open* **3**, e205873 (2020).

36. Pifer, R. Why are women more likely to use telehealth? *Healthcare Dive.* https://www.healthcaredive.com/news/women-more-likely-telehealth-patients-providers-covid-19-pandemic/608153/ (2021).

37. Kalmoe, M. C., Chapman, M. B., Gold, J. A. & Giedinghagen, A. M. Physician suicide: a call to action. *Mo. Med.* **116**, 211–216 (2019).

38. Holder, S. M., Peterson, E. R., Stephens, R. & Crandall, L. A. Stigma in mental health at the macro and micro levels: implications for mental health consumers and professionals. *Community Ment. Health J.* **55**, 369–374 (2019).

39. Lo, J. *et al.* Telehealth has played an outsized role meeting mental health needs during the COVID-19 pandemic. *KFF.* https://www.kff.org/coronavirus-covid-19/issue-brief/telehealth-has-played-an-outsized-role-meeting-mental-health-needs-during-the-covid-19-pandemic/ (2022).

40. Quality of care. https://www.who.int/health-topics/quality-of-care.

41. Chou, V. B., Walker, N. & Kanyangarara, M. Estimating the global impact of poor quality of care on maternal and neonatal outcomes in 81 low- and middle-income countries: a modeling study. *PLoS Med.* **16**, e1002990 (2019).

42. Institute of Medicine (US) Committee on Quality of Health Care in America. *To Err is Human: Building a Safer Health System.* (National Academies Press (US)).

43. Institute of Medicine (US) Committee on Quality of Health Care in America. *Crossing the Quality Chasm: A New Health System for the 21st Century.* (National Academies Press (US)).

44. Leapfrog group releases new hospital safety grades, marking 10th anniversary. Leapfrog. https://www.leapfroggroup.org/news-events/leapfrog-group-releases-new-hospital-safety-grades-marking-10th-anniversary (2022).

45. Reed, M. *et al.* Treatment and follow-up care associated with patient-scheduled primary care telemedicine and in-person visits in a large integrated health system. *JAMA Netw Open* **4**, e2132793 (2021).

46. Li, J.-P. O. *et al.* Safety of video-based telemedicine compared to in-person triage in emergency ophthalmology during COVID-19. *EClinicalMedicine* **34**, 100818 (2021).

47. Levine, D. M. *et al.* Remote vs in-home physician visits for hospital-level care at home: a randomized clinical trial. *JAMA Netw Open* **5**, e2229067 (2022).

48. Haque, M., Sartelli, M., McKimm, J. & Abu Bakar, M. Health care-associated infections—an overview. *Infect. Drug Resist.* **11**, 2321–2333 (2018).

49. Segal, J. B., Dukhanin, V. & Davis, S. Telemedicine in primary care: qualitative work towards a framework for appropriate use. *J. Am. Board Fam. Med.* **35**, 507–516 (2022).

50. Schlief, M. *et al.* Synthesis of the evidence on what works for whom in telemental health: rapid realist review. *Interact. J. Med. Res.* **11**, e38239 (2022).

51. Eichberg, D. G. *et al.* Telemedicine in neurosurgery: lessons learned from a systematic review of the literature for the COVID-19 era and beyond. *Neurosurgery* **88**, E1–E12 (2020).

52. Baughman, D. J. *et al.* Comparison of quality performance measures for patients receiving in-person vs telemedicine primary care in a large integrated health system. *JAMA Netw Open* **5**, e2233267 (2022).

53. Tchero, H. *et al.* Clinical effectiveness of telemedicine in diabetes mellitus: a meta-analysis of 42 randomized controlled trials. *Telemed. J. E. Health.* **25**, 569–583 (2019).

54. Borries, T. M. *et al.* The impact of telemedicine on patient self-management processes and clinical outcomes for patients with Types I or II diabetes mellitus in the United States: a scoping review. *Diabetes Metab. Syndr.* **13**, 1353–1357 (2019).

55. Demaerschalk, B. M. *et al.* Assessment of clinician diagnostic concordance with video telemedicine in the integrated multispecialty practice at Mayo Clinic during the beginning of COVID-19 pandemic from March to June 2020. *JAMA Netw Open* **5**, e2229958 (2022).

56. Junkins, A. *et al.* Feasibility, acceptability, and preliminary impact of telemedicine-administered cognitive behavioral therapy for adherence and depression among African American women living with HIV in the rural South. *J. Health Psychol.* **26**, 2730–2742 (2021).

57. Arsenault-Lapierre, G. *et al.* Hospital-at-home interventions vs in-hospital stay for patients with chronic disease who present to the emergency department: a systematic review and meta-analysis. *JAMA Netw Open* **4**, e2111568 (2021).

58. Chen, L. *et al.* Telemedicine in chronic wound management: systematic review and meta-analysis. *JMIR Mhealth Uhealth* **8**, e15574 (2020).

59. Uppal, A. *et al.* Adoption of telemedicine for postoperative follow-up after inpatient cancer-related surgery. *JCO Oncol Pract* **18**, e1091–e1099 (2022).

60. Xu, H., Granger, B. B., Drake, C. D., Peterson, E. D. & Dupre, M. E. Effectiveness of telemedicine visits in reducing 30-day readmissions among patients with heart failure during the COVID-19 pandemic. *J. Am. Heart Assoc.* **11**, e023935 (2022).

61. O'Connor, M. *et al.* Using telehealth to reduce all-cause 30-day hospital readmissions among heart failure patients receiving skilled home health services. *Appl. Clin. Inform.* **7**, 238–247 (2016).

62. Ben-Assa, E. *et al.* Is telemedicine an answer to reducing 30-day readmission rates post-acute myocardial infarction? *Telemed. J. E. Health.* **20**, 816–821 (2014).

63. Shah, V. V. *et al.* Association between in-person vs telehealth follow-up and rates of repeated hospital visits among patients seen in the emergency department. *JAMA Netw Open* **5**, e2237783 (2022).

64. Deschodt, M., Flamaing, J., Haentjens, P., Boonen, S. & Milisen, K. Impact of geriatric consultation teams on clinical outcome in acute hospitals: a systematic review and meta-analysis. *BMC Med.* **11**, 48 (2013).

65. Humphreys, J. & Harman, S. Late referral to palliative care consultation service: length of stay and in-hospital mortality outcomes. *J Community Support Oncol* **12**, 129–136 (2014).

66. Mohr, N. M. *et al.* Emergency department telemedicine shortens rural time-to-provider and emergency department transfer times. *Telemed. J. E. Health.* **24**, 582–593 (2018).

67. Mitra, A. *et al.* Telemedicine in paediatric emergency care: a systematic review. *J. Telemed. Telecare* 1357633X211010106 (2021).

68. Hohman, J. A. *et al.* Use of direct-to-consumer telemedicine to access mental health services. *J. Gen. Intern. Med.* **37**, 2759–2767 (2022).

69. Mason, A. N. The most important telemedicine patient satisfaction dimension: patient-centered care. *Telemed. J. E. Health.* **28**, 1206–1214 (2022).

70. Silva-Cardoso, J. *et al.* The future of telemedicine in the management of heart failure patients. *Card Fail Rev* **7**, e11 (2021).

71. Welch, G., Balder, A. & Zagarins, S. Telehealth program for type 2 diabetes: usability, satisfaction, and clinical usefulness in an urban community health center. *Telemed. J. E. Health.* **21**, 395–403 (2015).

72. Banbury, A., Nancarrow, S., Dart, J., Gray, L. & Parkinson, L. Telehealth interventions delivering home-based support group videoconferencing: systematic review. *J. Med. Internet Res.* **20**, e25 (2018).

73. Knapp, A., Harst, L., Hager, S., Schmitt, J. & Scheibe, M. Use of patient-reported outcome measures and patient-reported experience measures within evaluation studies of telemedicine applications: systematic review. *J. Med. Internet Res.* **23**, e30042 (2021).

74. Subbiah, I. M. *et al.* Association between telehealth and adherence with patient-reported outcomes (PRO)-based remote symptom monitoring among adolescent/young adults (AYA), middle age, and older adults with cancer. *J. Clin. Orthod.* **40**, 1513–1513 (2022).

75. Arora, M. *et al.* Cost-effectiveness analysis of telephone-based support for the management of pressure ulcers in people with spinal cord injury in India and Bangladesh. *Spinal Cord* **55**, 1071–1078 (2017).

76. Nguyen, H. V. *et al.* cost-effectiveness of a national telemedicine diabetic retinopathy screening program in Singapore. *Ophthalmology* **123**, 2571–2580 (2016).

77. Bernard, L. *et al.* Management of patients with rheumatoid arthritis by telemedicine: connected monitoring. A randomized controlled trial. *Joint Bone Spine* **89**, 105368 (2022).

78. Hays, R. D. & Skootsky, S. A. Patient experience with in-person and telehealth visits before and during the COVID-19 pandemic at a large integrated health system in the United States. *J. Gen. Intern. Med.* **37**, 847–852 (2022).

79. Gotthardt, C. J. *et al.* Patient satisfaction with care providers during the COVID-19 pandemic: an analysis of consumer assessment of health-care providers and systems survey scores for in-person and telehealth encounters at an academic medical center. *Telemed. J. E. Health.* (2023) doi:10.1089/tmj.2022.0460.

80. Goharinejad, S., Hajesmaeel-Gohari, S., Jannati, N., Goharinejad, S. & Bahaadinbeigy, K. Review of systematic reviews in the field of tele-medicine. *Med. J. Islam. Repub. Iran* **35**, 184 (2021).

81. Orlando, J. F., Beard, M. & Kumar, S. Systematic review of patient and caregivers' satisfaction with telehealth videoconferencing as a mode of service delivery in managing patients' health. *PLoS One* **14**, e0221848 (2019).

82. Kruse, C. S. *et al.* Telehealth and patient satisfaction: a systematic review and narrative analysis. *BMJ Open* **7**, e016242 (2017).

83. Pogorzelska, K. & Chlabicz, S. Patient satisfaction with telemedicine during the COVID-19 pandemic—A systematic review. *Int. J. Environ. Res. Public Health* **19** (2022).

84. Rapid growth in telehealth for cancer care. National Cancer Institute. https://www.cancer.gov/news-events/cancer-currents-blog/2022/pandemic-telehealth-surge-cancer-care (2022).

85. Patel, K. B. *et al.* Estimated indirect cost savings of using telehealth among nonelderly patients with cancer. *JAMA Netw Open* **6**, e2250211 (2023).

86. Nguyen, M., Waller, M., Pandya, A. & Portnoy, J. A Review of patient and provider satisfaction with telemedicine. *Curr. Allergy Asthma Rep.* **20**, 72 (2020).

87. Young, K., Gupta, A. & Palacios, R. Impact of telemedicine in pediatric postoperative care. *Telemed. J. E. Health.* **25**, 1083–1089 (2019).

88. Uemoto, Y. *et al.* Efficacy of telemedicine using videoconferencing systems in outpatient care for patients with cancer: a systematic review and meta-analysis. *JCO Clin Cancer Inform* **6**, e2200084 (2022).

89. Mohanty, A. *et al.* Ambulatory neurosurgery in the COVID-19 era: patient and provider satisfaction with telemedicine. *Neurosurg. Focus* **49**, E13 (2020).

90. Lanier, K., Kuruvilla, M. & Shih, J. Patient satisfaction and utilization of telemedicine services in allergy: an institutional survey. *J. Allergy Clin. Immunol. Pract.* **9**, 484–486 (2021).

91. Bagchi, A. D. *et al.* Comfort with telehealth among residents of an underserved urban area. *J. Prim. Care Community Health* **13**, 21501319221119692 (2022).

92. Hafeez, K. *et al.* Patient preference for virtual versus in-person visits in neuromuscular clinical practice. *Muscle Nerve* **66**, 142–147 (2022).

93. Welch, B. M., Harvey, J., O'Connell, N. S. & McElligott, J. T. Patient preferences for direct-to-consumer telemedicine services: a nationwide survey. *BMC Health Serv. Res.* **17**, 784 (2017).

94. McCoyd, J. L. M., Curran, L., Candelario, E. & Findley, P. "There is just a different energy": changes in the therapeutic relationship with the telehealth transition. *Clin. Soc. Work J.* **50**, 325–336 (2022).

95. Orrange, S., Patel, A., Mack, W. J. & Cassetta, J. Patient satisfaction and trust in telemedicine during the COVID-19 pandemic: retrospective observational study. *JMIR Hum Factors* **8**, e28589 (2021).

96. Ftouni, R., AlJardali, B., Hamdanieh, M., Ftouni, L. & Salem, N. Challenges of telemedicine during the COVID-19 pandemic: a systematic review. *BMC Med. Inform. Decis. Mak.* **22**, 207 (2022).

97. Doximity's new report finds adoption of telemedicine growing, majority of patients plan for virtual care post-pandemic. https://press.doximity.com/articles/doximity-s-new-report-finds-adoption-of-telemedicine-growing-majority-of-patients-plan-for-virtual-care-post-pandemic.

98. Sorensen, M. J., Bessen, S., Danford, J., Fleischer, C. & Wong, S. L. Telemedicine for surgical consultations—Pandemic response or here to stay?: a report of public perceptions. *Ann. Surg.* **272**, e174–e180 (2020).

99. Dhahri, A. A., Iqbal, M. R. & Pardoe, H. Agile application of video telemedicine during the COVID-19 pandemic. *Cureus* **12**, e11320 (2020).

100. Andreadis, K. *et al.* Telemedicine impact on the patient-provider relationship in primary care during the COVID-19 pandemic. *Med. Care* **61**, S83–S88 (2023).

101. Zhang, X. *et al.* Measuring telehealth visit length and schedule adherence using videoconferencing data. *Telemed. J. E. Health.* **28**, 976–984 (2022).

102. Vitto, C. *et al.* Teaching toolbox: breaking bad news with virtual technology in the time of COVID. *J. Cancer Educ.* **37**, 1429–1432 (2022).

103. Wolf, I., Waissengrin, B. & Pelles, S. Breaking bad news via telemedicine: a new challenge at times of an epidemic. *Oncologist* **25**, e879–e880 (2020).

104. Smrke, A. *et al.* Telemedicine during the COVID-19 pandemic: impact on care for rare cancers. *JCO Glob Oncol* **6**, 1046–1051 (2020).

105. McCabe, H. M. *et al.* What matters to us: impact of telemedicine during the pandemic in the care of patients with sarcoma across Scotland. *JCO Glob Oncol* **7**, 1067–1073 (2021).

106. Murphy, A., Kirby, A., Lawlor, A., Drummond, F. J. & Heavin, C. Mitigating the impact of the COVID-19 pandemic on adult cancer patients through telehealth adoption: a systematic review. *Sensors* **22**, (2022).

107. Johnson, B. A. *et al.* The new normal? Patient satisfaction and usability of telemedicine in breast cancer care. *Ann. Surg. Oncol.* **28**, 5668–5676 (2021).

108. Anderson, K., Coskun, R., Jimenez, P. & Omurtag, K. Satisfaction with new patient telehealth visits for reproductive endocrinology patients in the era of COVID-19. *J. Assist. Reprod. Genet.* **39**, 1571–1576 (2022).

109. Andrews, E., Berghofer, K., Long, J., Prescott, A. & Caboral-Stevens, M. Satisfaction with the use of telehealth during COVID-19: an integrative review. *Int J Nurs Stud Adv* **2**, 100008 (2020).

110. Mojdehbakhsh, R. P., Rose, S., Peterson, M., Rice, L. & Spencer, R. A quality improvement pathway to rapidly increase telemedicine services in a gynecologic oncology clinic during the COVID-19 pandemic with patient satisfaction scores and environmental impact. *Gynecol Oncol Rep* **36**, 100708 (2021).

111. Ebbert, J. O. *et al.* Patient preferences for telehealth services in a large multispecialty practice. *J. Telemed. Telecare* **29**, 298–303 (2023).

112. Predmore, Z. S., Roth, E., Breslau, J., Fischer, S. H. & Uscher-Pines, L. Assessment of patient preferences for telehealth in post-COVID-19 pandemic health care. *JAMA Netw Open* **4**, e2136405 (2021).

113. Rossini, A., Parente, A. & Howell, B. Perceptions of telehealth among commercial members who responded to a patient-experience survey during the onset of the Coronavirus-19 pandemic. *Telemed. J. E. Health.* **28**, 551–557 (2022).

114. Ohlstein, J. F., Ahmed, O. G., Garner, J. & Takashima, M. Telemedicine in otolaryngology in the COVID-19 era: a year out. *Cureus* **13**, e20794 (2021).

115. Anjana, R. M. *et al.* Acceptability and utilization of newer technologies and effects on glycemic control in type 2 diabetes: lessons learned from lockdown. *Diabetes Technol. Ther.* **22**, 527–534 (2020).

116. Bernocchi, P. *et al.* Home-based telesurveillance and rehabilitation after stroke: a real-life study. *Top. Stroke Rehabil.* **23**, 106–115 (2016).

117. Deshpande, A. *et al.* Asynchronous telehealth: a scoping review of analytic studies. *Open Med.* **3**, e69–91 (2009).

118. Aashima, Nanda, M. & Sharma, R. A review of patient satisfaction and experience with telemedicine: a virtual solution during and beyond COVID-19 pandemic. *Telemedicine and e-Health* **27**, 1325–1331 (2021).

119. Triemstra, J. D. & Lowery, L. Prevalence, predictors, and the financial impact of missed appointments in an academic adolescent clinic. *Cureus* **10**, e3613 (2018).

120. Adepoju, O. E. *et al.* Transition to telemedicine and its impact on missed appointments in community-based clinics. *Ann. Med.* **54**, 98–107 (2022).

121. Drerup, B., Espenschied, J., Wiedemer, J. & Hamilton, L. Reduced no-show rates and sustained patient satisfaction of telehealth during the COVID-19 pandemic. *Telemed. J. E. Health.* **27**, 1409–1415 (2021).

122. Donelan, K. *et al.* Patient and clinician experiences with telehealth for patient follow-up care. *Am. J. Manag. Care* **25**, 40–44 (2019).

123. Khairat, S. *et al.* Evaluation of patient experience during virtual and in-person urgent care visits: time and cost analysis. *J Patient Exp* **8**, 2374373520981487 (2021).

124. Patel, B. *et al.* Using a real-time locating system to evaluate the impact of telemedicine in an emergency department during COVID-19: observational study. *J. Med. Internet Res.* **23**, e29240 (2021).

125. Breton, M. *et al.* Telehealth challenges during COVID-19 as reported by primary healthcare physicians in Quebec and Massachusetts. *BMC Fam. Pract.* **22**, 192 (2021).

126. Cohen, T. N., Choi, E., Kanji, F. F., Scott, V. C. S. & Eilber, K. S. Patient and provider experience with telemedicine in a urology practice: identifying opportunities for improvement. *Practice* (2021) doi:10.1097/UPJ.0000000000000221.

127. Sarpong, N. O. *et al.* Reduction in hospital length of stay and increased utilization of telemedicine during the "return-to-normal" period of the COVID-19 pandemic does not adversely influence early clinical outcomes in patients undergoing total hip replacement: a case-control study. *Acta Orthop.* **93**, 528–533 (2022).

128. Rademacher, N. J. *et al.* Use of telemedicine to screen patients in the emergency department: matched cohort study evaluating efficiency and patient safety of telemedicine. *JMIR Med Inform* **7**, e11233 (2019).

129. Brunner-La Rocca, H.-P. *et al.* Reasons for readmission after hospital discharge in patients with chronic diseases-Information from an international dataset. *PLoS One* **15**, e0233457 (2020).

130. Lo, Y.-T., Chang, C.-M., Chen, M.-H., Hu, F.-W. & Lu, F.-H. Factors associated with early 14-day unplanned hospital readmission: a matched case-control study. *BMC Health Serv. Res.* **21**, 870 (2021).

131. Eustache, J., El-Kefraoui, C., Ekmekjian, T., Latimer, E. & Lee, L. Do postoperative telemedicine interventions with a communication feature reduce emergency department visits and readmissions?—a systematic review and meta-analysis. *Surg. Endosc.* **35**, 5889–5904 (2021).

132. McKissick, H. D., Cady, R. G., Looman, W. S. & Finkelstein, S. M. The impact of telehealth and care coordination on the number and type of clinical visits for children with medical complexity. *J. Pediatr. Health Care* **31**, 452–458 (2017).

133. Barnett, T. E. *et al.* The effectiveness of a care coordination home telehealth program for veterans with diabetes mellitus: a 2-year follow-up. *Am. J. Manag. Care* **12**, 467–474 (2006).

134. Ohl, M. *et al.* Mixed-methods evaluation of a telehealth collaborative care program for persons with HIV infection in a rural setting. *J. Gen. Intern. Med.* **28**, 1165–1173 (2013).

135. The complexities of physician supply and demand: projections from 2019 to 2034. Digital Collections, National Library of Medicine. http://resource.nlm.nih.gov/9918417887306676.

136. American Medical Association. Burnout benchmark: 28% unhappy with current health care job. *American Medical Association*. https://www.ama-assn.org/practice-management/physician-health/burnout-benchmark-28-unhappy-current-health-care-job (2022).

137. Shanafelt, T. D. *et al.* Changes in burnout and satisfaction with work-life integration in physicians during the first 2 years of the COVID-19 pandemic. *Mayo Clin. Proc.* **97**, 2248–2258 (2022).

138. Saiyed, S., Nguyen, A. & Singh, R. Physician perspective and key satisfaction indicators with rapid telehealth adoption during the coro-

navirus disease 2019 pandemic. *Telemed. J. E. Health.* **27**, 1225–1234 (2021).

139. COVID-19 healthcare coalition. COVID-19 Healthcare Coalition. https://c19hcc.org/telehealth/.

140. Malouff, T. D. *et al.* Physician satisfaction with telemedicine during the COVID-19 pandemic: the Mayo Clinic Florida experience. *Mayo Clin Proc Innov Qual Outcomes* **5**, 771–782 (2021).

141. American Medical Association. AMA digital health care 2022 study findings. American Medical Association. https://www.ama-assn.org/about/research/ama-digital-health-care-2022-study-findings (2022).

142. Park, H.-Y., Kwon, Y.-M., Jun, H.-R., Jung, S.-E. & Kwon, S.-Y. Satisfaction survey of patients and medical staff for telephone-based telemedicine during hospital closing due to COVID-19 transmission. *Telemed. J. E. Health.* **27**, 724–732 (2021).

143. Cordina, J., Fowkes, J., Malani, R. & Medford-Davis, L. Patients love telehealth—physicians are not so sure. https://www.mckinsey.com/industries/healthcare-systems-and-services/our-insights/patients-love-telehealth-physicians-are-not-so-sure (2022).

144. De Hert, S. Burnout in healthcare workers: prevalence, impact and preventative strategies. *Local Reg. Anesth.* **13**, 171–183 (2020).

145. Singh, R., Volner, K. & Marlowe, D. *Provider Burnout.* (StatPearls Publishing, 2022).

146. The complexities of physician supply and demand: projections from 2019 to 2034. Digital Collections, National Library of Medicine. https://digirepo.nlm.nih.gov/catalog/nlm:nlmuid-9918417887306676-pdf.

147. Thomas Craig, K. J., Willis, V. C., Gruen, D., Rhee, K. & Jackson, G. P. The burden of the digital environment: a systematic review on

organization-directed workplace interventions to mitigate physician burnout. *J. Am. Med. Inform. Assoc.* **28**, 985–997 (2021).

148. Garber, K. & Gustin, T. Telehealth education: impact on provider experience and adoption. *Nurse Educ.* **47**, 75–80 (2022).

149. Perry, K., Gold, S. & Shearer, E. M. Identifying and addressing mental health providers' perceived barriers to clinical video telehealth utilization. *J. Clin. Psychol.* **76**, 1125–1134 (2020).

150. Birkhäuer, J. *et al.* Trust in the health care professional and health outcome: a meta-analysis. *PLoS One* **12**, e0170988 (2017).

151. Elliott, T., Tong, I., Sheridan, A. & Lown, B. A. Beyond convenience: patients' perceptions of physician interactional skills and compassion via telemedicine. *Mayo Clin Proc Innov Qual Outcomes* **4**, 305–314 (2020).

152. Sperandeo, R. *et al.* Exploring the question: "Does empathy work in the same way in online and in-person therapeutic settings?" *Front. Psychol.* **12**, 671790 (2021).

153. Sakumoto, M. & Krug, S. Enhancing digital empathy and reimagining the telehealth experience. *THMT* (2021) doi:10.30953/tmt.v6.304.

154. Turner, A. P., Sloan, A. P., Kivlahan, D. R. & Haselkorn, J. K. Telephone counseling and home telehealth monitoring to improve medication adherence: results of a pilot trial among individuals with multiple sclerosis. *Rehabil. Psychol.* **59**, 136–146 (2014).

155. Winegard, B., Miller, E. G. & Slamon, N. B. Use of telehealth in pediatric palliative care. *Telemed. J. E. Health.* **23**, 938–940 (2017).

156. Kotsen, C. *et al.* Rapid scaling up of telehealth treatment for tobacco-dependent cancer patients during the COVID-19 outbreak in New York City. *Telemed. J. E. Health.* **27**, 20–29 (2021).

157. Molfenter, T. *et al.* Use of Telehealth in mental health (MH) services during and after COVID-19. *Community Ment. Health J.* **57**, 1244–1251 (2021).

158. Mark, T. L. *et al.* Addiction treatment and telehealth: review of efficacy and provider insights during the COVID-19 pandemic. *Psychiatr. Serv.* **73**, 484–491 (2022).

159. Project ECHO. https://www.ahrq.gov/patient-safety/settings/multiple/project-echo/index.html.

160. Gomez, T., Anaya, Y. B., Shih, K. J. & Tarn, D. M. A qualitative study of primary care physicians' experiences with telemedicine during COVID-19. *J. Am. Board Fam. Med.* **34**, S61–S70 (2021).

161. Croymans Daniel, Hurst Ian & Han Maria. Telehealth: the right care, at the right time, via the right medium. *Catalyst non-issue content* doi:10.1056/CAT.20.0564.

162. Benziger, C. P., Huffman, M. D., Sweis, R. N. & Stone, N. J. The telehealth ten: a guide for a patient-assisted virtual physical examination. *Am. J. Med.* **134**, 48–51 (2021).

163. Noel, K. & Fabus, R. *Telehealth—E-Book: Incorporating Interprofessional Practice for Healthcare Professionals in the 21st Century.* (Elsevier Health Sciences, 2022).

164. Conduct a telehealth physical exam. https://telehealth.hhs.gov/providers/preparing-patients-for-telehealth/telehealth-physical-exam/.

165. How to administer a virtual physical Exam. Stanford Department of Medicine, News. https://medicine.stanford.edu/news/current-news/standard-news/virtual-physical-exam.html.

166. Calloway, S., Guenther, J. & Merrill, E. 5-step guide for performing physical exams via telehealth. Preprint at https://www.clinicaladvisor.

com/home/topics/practice-management-information-center/5-step-guide-physical-exam-via-telehealth/2/ (2021).

167. Telehealth. https://shop.elsevier.com/books/telehealth/noel/978-0-7020-8423-2.

168. Sikka, N. *A Practical Guide to Emergency Telehealth*. (Oxford University Press, 2021).

169. Manuelyan, K., Shahid, M., Vassilev, V., Drenovska, K. & Vassileva, S. Direct patient-to-physician teledermatology: not a flash in the pan(demic). *Clin. Dermatol.* **39**, 45–51 (2021).

170. Broffman, L., Barnes, M., Stern, K. & Westergren, A. Evaluating the quality of asynchronous versus synchronous virtual care in patients with erectile dysfunction: retrospective cohort study. *JMIR Form Res* **6**, e32126 (2022).

171. Nguyen, O. T. *et al.* Impact of asynchronous electronic communication-based visits on clinical outcomes and health care delivery: systematic review. *J. Med. Internet Res.* **23**, e27531 (2021).

172. Ellimoottil, C., An, L., Moyer, M., Sossong, S. & Hollander, J. E. Challenges and opportunities faced by large health systems implementing telehealth. *Health Aff.* **37**, 1955–1959 (2018).

173. Narasimha, S. *et al.* An Investigation of the usability issues of home-based video telemedicine systems with geriatric patients. *Proc. Hum. Fact. Ergon. Soc. Annu. Meet.* **60**, 1804–1808 (2016).

174. Scott Kruse, C. *et al.* Evaluating barriers to adopting telemedicine worldwide: a systematic review. *J. Telemed. Telecare* **24**, 4–12 (2018).

175. Almathami, H. K. Y., Win, K. T. & Vlahu-Gjorgievska, E. Barriers and facilitators that influence telemedicine-based, real-time, online consultation at patients' homes: systematic literature review. *J. Med. Internet Res.* **22**, e16407 (2020).

176. M. A. L. How to get to know your users. *Smashing Magazine.* https://www.smashingmagazine.com/2018/06/how-to-get-to-know-your-users/ (2018).

177. Jackson, S. Telehealth failure a cautionary tale for U.S. Fierce Healthcare. https://www.fiercehealthcare.com/it/telehealth-failure-a-cautionary-tale-for-u-s (2012).

178. Hards, S. The ongoing cost of the NYY telehealth project exposed (UK). https://telecareaware.com/the-ongoing-cost-of-the-nyy-telehealth-project-exposed-uk/.

179. Chike-Harris, K. E., Durham, C., Logan, A., Smith, G. & DuBose-Morris, R. Integration of telehealth education into the health care provider curriculum: a review. *Telemed. J. E. Health.* **27**, 137–149 (2021).

180. Jiménez-Rodríguez, D. *et al.* Increase in video consultations during the COVID-19 pandemic: healthcare professionals' perceptions about their implementation and adequate management. *Int. J. Environ. Res. Public Health* **17**, (2020).

181. Shaver, J. The state of telehealth before and after the COVID-19 pandemic. *Prim. Care* **49**, 517–530 (2022).

182. Lawrence, K. *et al.* Building telemedicine capacity for trainees during the novel coronavirus outbreak: a case study and lessons learned. *J. Gen. Intern. Med.* **35**, 2675–2679 (2020).

183. Rutledge, C. M. *et al.* Telehealth and eHealth in nurse practitioner training: current perspectives. *Adv Med Educ Pract* **8**, 399–409 (2017).

184. Slovensky, D. J., Malvey, D. M. & Neigel, A. R. A model for mHealth skills training for clinicians: meeting the future now. *Mhealth* **3**, 24 (2017).

185. Telehealth competencies. AAMC. https://www.aamc.org/data-reports/report/telehealth-competencies.

186. Joshi, A. U. *et al.* Impact of emergency department tele-intake on left without being seen and throughput metrics. *Acad. Emerg. Med.* **27**, 139–147 (2020).

187. Wootton, R., Liu, J. & Bonnardot, L. Embedding telemedicine quality assurance within a large organisation. *European Research in Telemedicine* **5**, (2016).

188. Telehealth & quality assurance: the basics & the best practices. https://www.bugraptors.com/blog/telehealth-quality-assurance-the-basics-the-best-practices.

189. Sauro, J. & Lewis, J. R. Chapter 8—Standardized usability questionnaires. In *Quantifying the User Experience (Second Edition)* (eds. Sauro, J. & Lewis, J. R.) 185–248 (Morgan Kaufmann, 2016).

190. Reimagining prenatal care: a case for telemedicine. University of Utah Health. https://uofuhealth.utah.edu/notes/2019/06/reimagining-prenatal-care-case-telemedicine (2019).

191. Perrin, A. Mobile technology and home broadband 2021. Pew Research Center: Internet, Science & Tech. https://www.pewresearch.org/internet/2021/06/03/mobile-technology-and-home-broadband-2021/ (2021).

192. Charter Communications. What is the difference between a WiFi and Ethernet connection? https://enterprise.spectrum.com/support/faq/network/what-is-the-difference-between-wifi-and-ethernet-connection.html.

193. Global mobile traffic 2022. Statista. https://www.statista.com/statistics/277125/share-of-website-traffic-coming-from-mobile-devices/.

194. Cooper, T. How to tell if your internet is being throttled. Broadband-Now. https://broadbandnow.com/guides/am-i-being-throttled (2020).

195. Tracking COVID-19's impact on global internet performance (updated July 20). Ookla. https://www.ookla.com/articles/tracking-covid-19-impact-global-internet-performance (2020).

196. Office-based physician electronic health record adoption. https://www.healthit.gov/data/quickstats/office-based-physician-electronic-health-record-adoption.

197. Melnick, E. R. *et al.* The association between perceived electronic health record usability and professional burnout among US physicians. *Mayo Clin. Proc.* **95**, 476–487 (2020).

198. Ritchie, J. & Welch, B. Categorization of third-party apps in electronic health record app marketplaces: systematic search and analysis. *JMIR Med Inform* **8**, e16980 (2020).

199. AMA survey shows widespread enthusiasm for telehealth. American Medical Association. https://www.ama-assn.org/press-center/press-releases/ama-survey-shows-widespread-enthusiasm-telehealth.

200. Health Insurance Institute (New York &) N. Y. *Source Book of Health Insurance Data.* (Health Insurance Institute., 1982).

201. Appendix B. a brief history of managed care. https://www.ncd.gov/policy/appendix-b-brief-history-managed-care (2015).

202. Daley, J. Obama singles out Intermountain Healthcare as model system. https://www.ksl.com/article/7873613.

203. How corporate executives view rising health care cost and the role of government—findings. KFF. https://www.kff.org/report-section/how-corporate-executives-view-rising-health-care-cost-and-the-role-of-government-findings/ (2021).

204. Moon, M. Medicare matters: building on a record of accomplishments. *Health Care Financ. Rev.* **22**, 9–22 (2000).

205. Rudowitz, R., Garfield, R. & Hinton, E. 10 things to know about Medicaid: setting the facts straight. KFF. https://www.kff.org/medicaid/issue-brief/10-things-to-know-about-medicaid-setting-the-facts-straight/ (2019).

206. Chapter 8: Telehealth services and the Medicare program (June 2016 report). https://www.medpac.gov/document/http-www-medpac-gov-docs-default-source-reports-chapter-8-telehealth-services-and-the-medicare-program-june-2016-report-pdf/.

207. Harju, A. & Neufeld, J. The impact of the Medicaid expansion on telemental health utilization in four Midwestern States. *Telemed. J. E. Health.* **27**, 1260–1267 (2021).

208. Adler-Milstein, J., Kvedar, J. & Bates, D. W. Telehealth among US hospitals: several factors, including state reimbursement and licensure policies, influence adoption. *Health Aff.* **33**, 207–215 (2014).

209. 2021-12-30 15:27. https://www.hhs.gov/about/news/2021/12/03/new-hhs-study-shows-63-fold-increase-in-medicare-telehealth-utilization-during-pandemic.html.

210. Koma, W., Cubanski, J. & Neuman, T. Medicare and telehealth: coverage and use during the COVID-19 pandemic and options for the future. KFF. https://www.kff.org/medicare/issue-brief/medicare-and-telehealth-coverage-and-use-during-the-covid-19-pandemic-and-options-for-the-future/ (2021).

211. Chang, J. E. *et al.* Rapid transition to telehealth and the digital divide: implications for primary care access and equity in a post-COVID era. *Milbank Q.* **99**, 340–368 (2021).

212. Payán, D. D., Frehn, J. L., Garcia, L., Tierney, A. A. & Rodriguez, H. P. Telemedicine implementation and use in community health centers

during COVID-19: clinic personnel and patient perspectives. *SSM Qual Res Health* **2**, 100054 (2022).

213. Trump administration releases COVID-19 telehealth toolkit to accelerate state use of telehealth in Medicaid and CHIP. https://www.cms.gov/newsroom/press-releases/trump-administration-releases-covid-19-telehealth-toolkit-accelerate-state-use-telehealth-medicaid.

214. How the pandemic continues to shape Medicaid priorities: results from an annual Medicaid budget survey for state fiscal years 2022 and 2023—telehealth. KFF. https://www.kff.org/report-section/medicaid-budget-survey-for-state-fiscal-years-2022-and-2023-telehealth/ (2022).

215. United States. Government Accountability Office. *Medicaid: CMS Should Assess Effect of Increased Telehealth Use on Beneficiaries' Quality of Care: Report to Congressional Committees.* (United States Government Accountability Office, 2022).

216. Principles of health economics including: the notions of scarcity, supply and demand, distinctions between need and demand, opportunity cost, discounting, time horizons, margins, efficiency and equity. https://www.healthknowledge.org.uk/public-health-textbook/medical-sociology-policy-economics/4d-health-economics/principles-he.

217. Office of Public & Intergovernmental Affairs. Office of public and intergovernmental affairs. https://www.va.gov/opa/pressrel/pressrelease.cfm?id=546.

218. Mathews, C. P., Convoy, S., Heyworth, L. & Knisely, M. Evaluation of the use of telehealth video visits for veterans with chronic pain. *Pain Manag. Nurs.* **23**, 418–423 (2022).

219. Russo, J. E., McCool, R. R. & Davies, L. VA telemedicine: an analysis of cost and time savings. *Telemed. J. E. Health.* **22**, 209–215 (2016).

220. Egede, L. E., Dismuke, C. E., Walker, R. J., Acierno, R. & Frueh, B. C. Cost-effectiveness of behavioral activation for depression in older adult veterans: in-person care versus telehealth. *J. Clin. Psychiatry* **79**, (2018).

221. Painter, J. T., Fortney, J. C., Austen, M. A. & Pyne, J. M. Cost-effectiveness of telemedicine-based collaborative care for posttraumatic stress disorder. *Psychiatr. Serv.* **68**, 1157–1163 (2017).

222. Audit of TRICARE telehealth payments (DODIG-2022-047). Department of Defense Office of Inspector General. https://www.dodig.mil/reports.html/Article/2925081/audit-of-tricare-telehealth-payments-dodig-2022-047/ (2022).

223. Carroll, M. *et al.* Innovation in Indian healthcare: using health information technology to achieve health equity for American Indian and Alaska Native populations. *Perspect. Health Inf. Manag.* **8**, 1d (2011).

224. Home. https://www.internetforall.gov/.

225. Thomas, E. E. *et al.* Beyond forced telehealth adoption: a framework to sustain telehealth among allied health services. *J. Telemed. Telecare* 1357633X221074499 (2022).

226. Raj Westwood, A. Is hybrid telehealth model the next step for private healthcare in India? *Health. Serv. Insights* **14**, 11786329211043301 (2021).

227. Crouch, H. Exclusive: GP at Hand partner hits back at cherry picking concerns. Digital Health. https://www.digitalhealth.net/2018/04/exclusive-babylon-cherry-picking-concerns-not-justified/ (2018).

228. Babylon GP at Hand now fifth largest practice in England. GP. https://www.gponline.com/babylon-gp-hand-fifth-largest-practice-england/article/1593735 (2019).

229. Crouch, H. Patients and GPs gather for protest against GP at Hand. Digital Health. https://www.digitalhealth.net/2018/03/gp-at-hand-protests-east-london/ (2018).

230. Singapore's COVID breath tests give results within 2 minutes. Nikkei Asia. https://asia.nikkei.com/Spotlight/Coronavirus/Singapore-s-COVID-breath-tests-give-results-within-2-minutes (2021).

231. Richter, L. & Silberzahn, T. Germany's e-health infrastructure strengthens, but digital uptake is lagging. https://www.mckinsey.com/industries/life-sciences/our-insights/germanys-e-health-infrastructure-strengthens-but-digital-uptake-is-lagging (2020).

232. 2022 employer health benefits survey—section 1: cost of health insurance. KFF. https://www.kff.org/report-section/ehbs-2022-section-1-cost-of-health-insurance/ (2022).

233. Estimating the potential profit gains from lowering employee health care costs for America's largest companies. Baker Institute. https://www.bakerinstitute.org/research/estimating-potential-profit-gains-lowering-employee-health-care-costs-americas-largest.

234. Telemedicine. Congressional Budget Office. https://www.cbo.gov/publication/50680 (2015).

235. Ashwood, J. S., Mehrotra, A., Cowling, D. & Uscher-Pines, L. Direct-to-consumer telehealth may increase access to care but does not decrease spending. *Health Aff.* **36**, 485–491 (2017).

236. Centers for Medicare & Medicaid Services Center for Consumer Information and Insurance Oversight. *FAQs on Availability and Usage of Telehealth Services through Private Health Insurance Coverage in Response to Coronavirus Disease 2019 (COVID-19).* Preprint at https://www.cms.gov/files/document/faqs-telehealth-covid-19.pdf (2020).

237. Wicklund, E. Walmart expands telehealth services for employees in 3 states. mHealthIntelligence. https://mhealthintelligence.com/news/walmart-expands-telehealth-services-for-employees-in-3-states (2019).

238. 2021 employer health benefits survey—section 13: employer practices, telehealth and employer responses to the pandemic. KFF. https://www.kff.org/report-section/ehbs-2021-section-13-employer-practices-tele-health-and-employer-responses-to-the-pandemic/ (2021).

239. Johnston, B., Wheeler, L., Deuser, J. & Sousa, K. H. Outcomes of the Kaiser Permanente Tele-Home Health Research Project. *Arch. Fam. Med.* **9**, 40–45 (2000).

240. Johnston, B., Wheeler, L. & Deuser, J. Kaiser Permanente Medical Center's pilot Tele-Home Health Project. *Telemed. Today* **5**, 16–7, 19 (1997).

241. Cohen, R. A., Terlizzi, E. P. & Martinez, M. E. Home page. https://doi.org/.

242. DeMarco, J. Rate of workers enrolled in high-deductible health plans jumps for 8th year in row to record 55.7%. ValuePenguin. https://www.valuepenguin.com/high-deductible-health-plan-study (2023).

243. Landi, H. Amazon scoops up primary care company One Medical in deal valued at $3.9B. Fierce Healthcare. https://www.fiercehealthcare.com/health-tech/amazon-shells-out-39b-primary-care-startup-one-medical (2022).

244. Massive growth in expenses & rising inflation fuel financial challenges for America's hospitals & health systems. American Hospital Association. https://www.aha.org/guidesreports/2022-04-22-massive-growth-expenses-and-rising-inflation-fuel-continued-financial.

245. Vollers, A. C. Doctors struggle to pay bills in pandemic and telemedicine isn't saving them. https://www.al.com/news/2020/04/doctors-

struggle-pay-bills-in-pandemic-and-telemedicine-isnt-saving-them.
html (2020).

246. Spaulding, R., Belz, N., DeLurgio, S. & Williams, A. R. Cost savings
of telemedicine utilization for child psychiatry in a rural Kansas
community. *Telemed. J. E. Health.* **16**, 867–871 (2010).

247. Buvik, A. *et al.* Cost-effectiveness of telemedicine in remote orthopedic
consultations: randomized controlled trial. *J. Med. Internet Res.* **21**,
e11330 (2019).

248. Ma, Y. *et al.* Post-operative telephone review is safe and effective: prospective study—Monash outpatient review by phone trial. *ANZ J. Surg.*
88, 434–439 (2018).

249. *2022 MGMA Data Report—Patient Access and Value-Based
Outcomes Amid the Great Attrition.* https://www.mgma.com/data/
landing-pages/2022-mgma-data-dive-better-performers-report.

250. Yilmaz, S. K., Horn, B. P., Fore, C. & Bonham, C. A. An economic
cost analysis of an expanding, multi-state behavioural telehealth intervention. *J. Telemed. Telecare* **25**, 353–364 (2019).

251. Kovács, G., Somogyvári, Z., Maka, E. & Nagyjánosi, L. Bedside ROP
screening and telemedicine interpretation integrated to a neonatal
transport system: economic aspects and return on investment analysis.
Early Hum. Dev. **106-107**, 1–5 (2017).

252. Hafner, M., Yerushalmi, E., Dufresne, E. & Gkousis, E. *Greater
Adoption of Telemedicine Could Offer Economic and Social Benefits for
Canada.* (RAND Corporation, 2021).

253. Adepoju, O. E., Angelocci, T. & Matuk-Villazon, O. Increased revenue
from averted missed appointments following telemedicine adoption
at a large federally qualified health center. *Health Serv Insights* **15**,
11786329221125409 (2022).

254. Zocchi, M., Uscher-Pines, L., Ober, A. & Kapinos, K. *Costs of Maintaining a High-Volume Telemedicine Program in Community Health Centers*. (RAND Corporation, 2020).

255. Xiang, X. M. & Bernard, J. Telehealth in multiple sclerosis clinical care and research. *Curr. Neurol. Neurosci. Rep.* **21**, 14 (2021).

256. Lo, M. D. & Gospe, S. M., Jr. Telemedicine and child neurology. *J. Child Neurol.* **34**, 22–26 (2019).

257. Florida businesswoman pleads guilty to criminal health care and tax fraud charges and agrees to $20.3 million civil false claims act settlement. https://www.justice.gov/opa/pr/florida-businesswoman-pleads-guilty-criminal-health-care-and-tax-fraud-charges-and-agrees-203 (2021).

258. Federal agencies watching for Medicare abuse as telehealth expanded during the pandemic. SAI360. https://www.sai360.com/resources/grc/compliance-grc/watching-for-medicare-abuse-as-telehealth-use-expands-during-the-pandemic (2022).

259. Muchmore, S. & Pifer, R. $6B fraud bust includes numerous telehealth schemes. Healthcare Dive. https://www.healthcaredive.com/news/6b-fraud-bust-includes-numerous-telehealth-schemes/586220/ (2020).

260. Burlington county doctor sentenced to 33 months in prison for role in $24 million telemedicine compounded medication scheme. https://www.justice.gov/usao-nj/pr/burlington-county-doctor-sentenced-33-months-prison-role-24-million-telemedicine (2021).

261. U.S. Attorney announces criminal and civil enforcement actions against medical practitioners for roles in telemedicine fraud schemes. https://www.justice.gov/usao-wdmi/pr/2021_0824_Happy_Clickers (2021).

262. Four people indicted in international telemedicine health care fraud kickback scheme. https://www.justice.gov/usao-nj/pr/four-people-

indicted-international-telemedicine-health-care-fraud-kickback-scheme (2021).

263. Special fraud alerts, bulletins, and other guidance. Office of Inspector General, Government Oversight, U.S. Department of Health and Human Services. https://oig.hhs.gov/compliance/alerts/ (2021).

264. Food, U.S., Administration, D. & Others. CFR-code of federal regulations title 21. Preprint at https://www.accessdata.fda.gov/scripts/cdrh/cfdocs/cfcfr/CFRSearch.cfm?CFRPart=1306 (2017).

265. Gliadkovskaya, A. Bicycle Health flies staff into Alabama to save hundreds of its patients from losing access to care under new law. Fierce Healthcare. https://www.fiercehealthcare.com/providers/bicycle-health-flies-physicians-alabama-maintain-patient-care-under-new-law (2022).

266. Vestal, C. As abortion pills take off, some states move to curb them. https://www.pewtrusts.org/en/research-and-analysis/blogs/stateline/2022/03/16/as-abortion-pills-take-off-some-states-move-to-curb-them (2022).

267. Sobel, L., Ramaswamy, A. & Salganicoff, A. The intersection of state and federal policies on access to medication abortion via telehealth. KFF. https://www.kff.org/womens-health-policy/issue-brief/the-intersection-of-state-and-federal-policies-on-access-to-medication-abortion-via-telehealth/ (2022).

268. Online prescribing. CCHP. https://www.cchpca.org/topic/online-prescribing/.

269. Blackstock, O. J., Shah, P. A., Haughton, L. J., Horvath, K. J. & Cunningham, C. O. HIV-infected women's perspectives on the use of the internet for social support: a potential role for online group-based interventions. *J. Assoc. Nurses AIDS Care* **26**, 411–419 (2015).

270. Green, S. M., Lockhart, E. & Marhefka, S. L. Advantages and disadvantages for receiving Internet-based HIV/AIDS interventions at home or at community-based organizations. *AIDS Care* **27**, 1304–1308 (2015).

271. Ornstein, C., Waldman, A. & Tigas, M. VA Midwest health care network (VISN 23). ProPublica. https://projects.propublica.org/hipaa/reports/b08c5b5f3b1e82face6849af638999450207a012.

272. Ornstein, C., Waldman, A. & Tigas, M. Tomah VA medical center. ProPublica. https://projects.propublica.org/hipaa/reports/f55b869c30a227bbcb4ea4c6e21090b66256ff4b.

273. Borisova, D. Zoom will owe you $15 after lawsuit for lying about encryption. PhoneArena. https://www.phonearena.com/news/Zoom-owes-you-20-after-lawsuit-for-lying-about-encryption_id134097 (2021).

274. Office for Civil Rights (OCR). Minimum necessary requirement. HHS.gov. https://www.hhs.gov/hipaa/for-professionals/privacy/guidance/minimum-necessary-requirement/index.html (2009).

275. Ornstein, C. Hospital to punish snooping on Spears. *Los Angeles Times* (2008).

276. Palmer, K. "Out of control": dozens of telehealth startups sent sensitive health information to Big Tech companies. The Markup. https://themarkup.org/pixel-hunt/2022/12/13/out-of-control-dozens-of-telehealth-startups-sent-sensitive-health-information-to-big-tech-companies.

277. McKeon, J. Telehealth companies under scrutiny for allegedly sharing health data with third-party advertisers. HealthITSecurity. https://healthitsecurity.com/news/telehealth-companies-under-scrutiny-for-allegedly-sharing-health-data-with-third-party-advertisers (2023).

278. HIPAA Journal. Cignet fined 4.3 m for HIPAA privacy rule violation. *HIPAA Journal.* https://www.hipaajournal.com/cignet-fined-4-3-m-for-hipaa-privacy-rule-violation/ (2011).

279. Thomas, G. Defending your data from the dark overlord. OncLive. https://www.chiefhealthcareexecutive.com/view/defending-your-data-from-the-dark-overlord (2018).

280. Weckler, A. HSE working to restore IT systems amid claims hackers demand $20m for stolen data. SundayWorld.com. https://www.sundayworld.com/news/irish-news/hse-working-to-restore-it-systems-amid-claims-hackers-demand-20m-for-stolen-data/40431150.html (2021).

281. Cullen, P. Cyberattack: HSE faces final bill of at least €100m. *Irish Times* (2021).

282. Bergal, J. Ransomware attacks on hospitals put patients at risk. https://www.pewtrusts.org/en/research-and-analysis/blogs/stateline/2022/05/18/ransomware-attacks-on-hospitals-put-patients-at-risk (2022).

283. The State of Ransomware in Healthcare 2022. SOPHOS. https://www.sophos.com/en-us/whitepaper/state-of-ransomware-in-healthcare.

284. HIPAA Journal. $475,000 settlement for delayed HIPAA breach notification. *HIPAA Journal.* https://www.hipaajournal.com/475000-settlement-delayed-hipaa-breach-notification-8640/ (2017).

285. Osborne, C. Data breach forces medical debt collector AMCA to file for bankruptcy protection. ZDNET. https://www.zdnet.com/article/medical-debt-collector-amca-files-for-bankruptcy-protection-after-data-breach/ (2019).

286. U.S. Department of Health & Human Services—Office for Civil Rights. https://ocrportal.hhs.gov/ocr/breach/breach_report.jsf.

287. Davis, J. Florida Orthopaedic reaches $4M settlement over 2020 health data theft. *SC Media.* https://www.scmagazine.com/analysis/ransomware/florida-orthopaedic-reaches-4m-settlement-over-2020-health-data-theft (2022).

288. Bischoff, P. How data breaches affect stock market share prices. Comparitech. https://www.comparitech.com/blog/information-security/data-breach-share-price-analysis/ (2019).

289. Doctor sentenced in Internet prescription case. https://www.almanacnews.com/news/2009/04/18/doctor-sentenced-in-internet-prescription-case (2009).

290. Teladoc, inc. V. Tex. Med. Bd., 1-15-CV-343 RP. https://casetext.com/case/teladoc-inc-v-tex-med-bd-1 (2015).

291. North Carolina State Board of Dental Examiners v. FTC. *Harvard Law Review.* https://harvardlawreview.org/print/vol-129/north-carolina-state-board-of-dental-examiners-v-ftc-2/ (2015).

292. Walters, E. Federal regulators take teladoc's side in medical board suit. *The Texas Tribune* (2016).

293. Davis, J. Teladoc drops Texas lawsuit as state adopts new telemedicine regulation. Healthcare IT News. https://www.healthcareitnews.com/news/teladoc-drops-texas-lawsuit-state-adopts-new-telemedicine-regulation (2017).

294. Appleby, J. Telehealth's limits: battle over state lines and licensing threatens patients' options. KFF Health News https://kffhealthnews.org/news/article/state-medical-licensing-rules-threatens-telehealth-patient-options/ (2021).

295. Federation of State Medical Boards. U.S. states and territories modifying requirements for telehealth in response to COVID-19. https://www.fsmb.org/siteassets/advocacy/pdf/states-waiving-licensure-requirements-for-telehealth-in-response-to-covid-19.pdf (2023).

296. Tedeschi, C. Ethical, legal, and social challenges in the development and implementation of disaster telemedicine. *Disaster Med. Public Health Prep.* **15**, 649–656 (2021).

297. Mehrotra, A., Nimgaonkar, A. & Richman, B. Telemedicine and Medical licensure - Potential paths for reform. *N. Engl. J. Med.* **384**, 687–690 (2021).

298. Becker, C. D., Dandy, K., Gaujean, M., Fusaro, M. & Scurlock, C. Legal perspectives on telemedicine part 1: legal and regulatory issues. *Perm. J.* **23**, (2019).

299. Welch, B. M. *et al.* Teleconsent: a novel approach to obtain informed consent for research. *Contemp Clin Trials Commun* **3**, 74–79 (2016).